THE END OF
THE GOLDEN AGE
OF GENERAL SURGERY

1870–2000

THE TRAINING AND PRACTICE OF A GENERAL
SURGEON IN THE LATE TWENTIETH CENTURY

BY

NIGEL KEITH MAYBURY

ISBN: 1499531370
ISBN 13: 9781499531374
Library of Congress Control Number: 2014908865
CreateSpace Independent Publishing Platform
North Charleston, South Carolina

To Sara, for her love

Contents

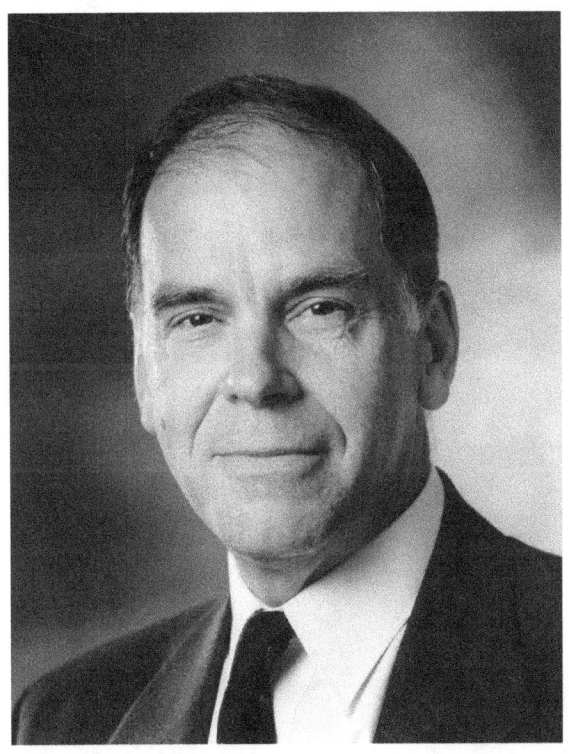

N. Keith Maybury, MA, DM, FRCS, FLS.
Photograph by Rayment Kirby, 1999.

Prologue

The "Golden Age of General Surgery" was approximately one hundred and thirty years long, lasting from about 1870 to 2000. It opened with the availability of general anaesthesia. This enabled surgeons for the first time to operate safely within the body cavities. This capability, coupled with trainee surgeons having to be resident in hospital to learn their craft during a long and arduous apprenticeship, produced general surgeons able to practise over a very broad field of expertise. Throughout this period, consultants had control over how they practised, which was usually referred to as "clinical freedom."

Some compounds capable of inducing numbness in a localised area were known in antiquity, but the modern era of anaesthetics was ushered in following the discovery of agents capable of providing reliable and reversible loss of consciousness in patients. This relieved the surgeon of the necessity to carry out an operation as fast as possible, in order to keep the inevitable agony to the minimum. This pain was graphically alluded to by Samuel Pepys in his *Diary* and was such that, following his operation for removal of a bladder stone by Thomas Hollier of St Thomas's and Bart's in 1657, he would thereafter hold an annual celebration commemorating his survival. Robert Liston (1794–1847), a famous Scottish surgeon, was described by a colleague in the preanaesthetic age as "the fastest knife in the West," as he was able to carry out amputation of a leg in two and a half minutes. The importance of speed was emphasised by Florence Nightingale, who stated after the Crimean War (1853–1856) that the risk of death (during an operation) was in direct ratio to the time that the operation lasted.

By using ether or chloroform, operations such as amputations could now be performed without undue haste. Robert Liston performed an amputation of a leg, with the patient under an ether general anaesthetic in 1846. Surgeons then began to contemplate complex and lengthy elective operations.

The three great body cavities, abdominal, thoracic, and cranial, could now be opened for the first time for preplanned elective surgery. This explosion of entirely new operations was the beginning of the golden age of the general surgeon. Arguably the greatest surgeon of this time was Theodor Billroth (1829–1894), who in Vienna carried out an oesophagectomy in 1871, a laryngectomy in 1873, and the first successful gastrectomy for cancer in 1881. Such operations were not immediately accepted by other surgeons or by the populace. After the death of one of his early gastrectomy patients, Billroth was stoned by an angry crowd and was lucky to escape. He survived to train a generation of outstanding surgeons. Amongst them was John B. Murphy, who returned to his native America, where he advocated surgery for acute appendicitis that subsequently became routine. Another was William S. Halsted, who instituted an early surgical residency programme based on Billroth's teaching methods. This residency programme was adopted in Great Britain and represented a true apprenticeship for house officers and registrars. Halsted performed the first gall-bladder operation in the United States in 1882 and developed the operation of radical mastectomy in the same year, which was named after him. This latter operation was not totally superseded until the mid-1970s, whereas all the other operations are still performed. Arguably the first time that the thorax was opened electively, and the patient survived, was following a partial lung resection for a tumour, carried out in 1884 by Kronlein in Zurich. Operations within the cranium came still later.

From the beginning of the golden age, it was not long before all parts of the body were coming within the remit of the general surgeon. As advances in treatment occurred, specialities were developed, initially still within general surgery, but with time these developed their own ethos and examinations. During the author's training from 1962 to 1980, general surgery still encompassed the whole gastro-intestinal tract, thoracic surgery (excluding cardiac surgery), urology, biliary surgery, pancreatic surgery, paediatric surgery, breast surgery, endocrine surgery, trauma surgery (including emergency neurosurgery), surgery of the acute abdomen, and vascular surgery.

The author describes his experience within this framework from his time as a medical student until his retirement as a consultant. Independence of practice continued until the late 1990s, when the way surgeons work gradually started to be radically changed. As the author's generation of general surgeons retired, their successors are specialists who focus on a single area of expertise due to the abandonment of the apprenticeship and the considerable shortening of the time spent training. This book is the story of the journey of one general surgeon's training and his subsequent experience and responsibilities as a consultant before the changes made the old mode of practise impossible. To write this book he was able to draw on detailed personal records kept over the years.

The old way of working during the last decades of the twentieth century had many advantages. Patients, both NHS and private, were routinely referred by their general practitioners to a surgeon by name. Thus, that surgeon had ownership of, and personal responsibility to, individual patients under his or her care. This continuity of care was reflected in the Consultant Contract of 1980, which in one succinct sentence clearly expressed, "A continuing clinical responsibility for patients in your charge." This duty was taken seriously. The consultant, whether on duty for new emergencies or not, expected to be informed of his or her patients' clinical problems by day or night.

During the last decades of the twentieth century, priority for patients to have operations was allocated by clinical urgency alone. There was no role at all for management in this, also there were no targets. All consultants were de facto equal in status and pay. This inverted pyramid in the career structure effectively meant that all consultants, including professors who were also consultants, had reached the top of their professional tree. This structure gave great job satisfaction and status to all consultants. Every consultant from that era would have been included as a "person with autonomous decision-taking powers" under the European Working Time Directive. That many consultants are not so designated in the twenty-first century NHS is significant.

The author recognises that change was inevitable and driven by many factors, including the rapid advances of science, engineering and electronics. During this time, there was an extraordinary increase in the sophistication of investigative internal imaging, including ultrasound, CT, and MRI scanners leading to three-dimensional images and PET scanners, for example. New and sophisticated instruments have increased the range of surgery carried out laparoscopically, and robotic surgery is now underway. More effective chemotherapy and radiotherapy has in some cases and diseases replaced the necessity for an operation at all. The genetic revolution has also only just begun and is expected to yield great advances.

Legal and management changes include the European Time Directive which has necessitated a total overhaul of training, especially a significant reduction in the length of time in training and the loss of the apprenticeship. The imposition of targets has distorted practice and given managers a great role in dictating priorities, curtailing the independence of surgeons. The percentage of the aged in the population has greatly increased and must be accommodated. With goodwill and hard work, a career in surgery should remain a rewarding, useful, and exciting way of life. Different solutions are needed for different times, and as these changes have occurred, surgery has transformed from being the art of medical science to the aplication of the technology of medical science. The author wishes his successors well but is grateful that he practised surgery when he did, before the golden age of the general surgeon closed.

Acknowledgements

I owe thanks to many people for their teaching, example, and friendship and apologise to those who have not been mentioned. I am grateful to: the late Canon Fredrick John Shirley, the charismatic but strict headmaster of the King's School, Canterbury; Mr John Wilson, philosopher, author, and sometime housemaster of Walpole House, where I and other boys flourished; Mr Percy O'Brien, who tutored me at Pembroke, giving brilliant insights into physiology; Dr Max Cowan, the meticulous anatomist who made the subject absorbing; Mr R. W. Nevin, dean of the medical school of St Thomas's Hospital, under whose benign tutelage and long experience I started my career in surgery; Professor Davis, professor of anatomy at St Thomas's Hospital Medical School and editor of *Gray's Anatomy*, which he made easy reading; Mr Frank Cockett, consultant surgeon at St Thomas's who was known to all as the "Ace," and whose introduction to private practise was memorable; Mr John Marsh, consultant general surgeon at Warwick Hospital, who taught me to operate and introduced me to the fascinating and broad sweep of his expertise; Mr William Slack, later knighted, consultant surgeon at the Middlesex Hospital and a kindly chief who introduced me to academic surgery; Professor Michael Hobsley, supervisor for my research and thesis, whose grasp of science was profound; Professor Peter Bell, later knighted, professor of surgery at Leicester University, who taught me vascular surgery and how to manage twin operating theatres to the great advantage of all; and Mr Michael Johnson, consultant surgeon at Leicester Royal Infirmary, from whom I learned the intricacies and delicacy of paediatric surgery.

My thanks go to Brian Livingstone, FRCS, whose friendship I value, who has read the document with many useful suggestions and corrections. I also thank my wife, Sara, who has always supported and encouraged me throughout my career, including the preparation and writing of this book, which has been gestating for ten years. However any opinions or errors are entirely mine.

CHAPTER 1:

An Undergraduate at Oxford, 1962-1966

At Pembroke College, in 1962, I benefitted from the prestigious tutorial system of teaching. It was an ancient system, based on personal tutorials between tutor and undergraduate and was usually held in the tutor's rooms in college. Each tutorial lasted an hour, and an essay that had been set the week before was presented. In my first year, I was given tutorials by both Dr Max Cowan and Mr Percy O'Brien at Pembroke. In my second and third years, I was tutored by Mr O'Brien and Dr Torrance at St John's, and finally in my fourth year by Dr Poole of Corpus Christi College.

Dr Cowan, a soft-spoken South African, was a neurophysiologist and an anatomist of meticulous and serious demeanour. He tutored in both these subjects. I was aware that all my tutors were scientists who were researching at the frontiers of their subjects. Having an hour a week of their time to discuss the work done for the essay meant that the work that went into the essay steadily increased as the weeks went by. As my understanding increased, there was an opportunity to discuss in depth the science behind the topic of the week. It was certainly very stimulating and kept the work interesting. Work, however, was never all-pervasive, and with good time management, there was time for other pursuits. Since the traditional role of the university was research, with teaching only as a by-product, the terms were short, there being three eight-week terms in the year. The result was that during six months of the year, the undergraduates were on vacation and then the dons could concentrate on their research without interruption. The undergraduates could also study and do other things in these vacations, especially as the summer vacation was four months long.

For one vacation, Dr Cowan borrowed my copy of the new edition of *Gray's Anatomy*, given to me by my father, and at the end of the vacation, I found the book placed in my pigeon hole in the college lodge, with a note exhorting me to make good use of the book. I did, although some years later. After I had gone down, Dr Cowan moved to the United States, where he eventually became the chief of the Federal Grant Organisation for Neurophysiology.

Mr O'Brien was my principal tutor. He was a short balding man who was always bursting with energy. He was the head of the biochemistry laboratory at the Radcliffe Infirmary. Not only a biochemist but a superb physiologist, he was my tutor in both subjects. He taught me how to organise my thoughts before making either an oral presentation or writing an essay, insisting on a logical flow of information and also that any written work was illustrated with relevant line drawings and graphs. If there was a tutorial with Mr O'Brian in the early evening before dinner in hall, he always offered a glass of sherry that would be sipped while discussing the 'queen of sciences': physiology. He always claimed that he could never remember names, and so he called all the men Willy and all the women Lizzy. In spite of this, he kept a very close eye on the progress of all his students. I greatly admired Mr O'Brien and have remained thankful for his inspired teaching. However, he could be irritating at times, and I did fall out with him some years later, for which I was sorry.

Mr O'Brien was a very practical man, and it was understood that he inspected his whole department every morning, including the lavatories. One day, he found the lavatories dirty and summoned the cleaning staff. When they were assembled, he cleaned the lavatories himself to demonstrate how it should be done. The lavatories were always spotless thereafter. Mr O'Brien was a man who led from the front. He always said he preferred his doctor of philosophy (DPhil) students to have second-class degrees (equivalent to a 2.1 nowadays). He claimed that those with first-class degrees rarely had an idea amongst them. This, of course, was a typical gross exaggeration. However, in the sixties, fewer than 5% of undergraduates were awarded a first-class degree at Oxford. In 2010, 25% of undergraduates were awarded a first. This represents significant grade inflation, and in spite of what was written in this paragraph about firsts, this inflation is unfair to the truly brilliant, who are denied their rightful recognition.

Mr O'Brien's own research had been directed to elucidating the molecular structure of haemoglobin. This molecule evolved to capture and hold oxygen safely in the red blood cells while transporting them to the tissues, where their powerful oxidation could be safely utilised. He was making progress in discovering the detail of this structure but lost the race to Dr Max Perutz. Years later, I heard a brilliant lecture given by Professor Perutz in Manchester on the comparative physiology of haemoglobin. Max Perutz was awarded the Nobel Prize for Chemistry in 1962 for his work on laying bare the structure of haemoglobin.

Dr Poole was a pathologist who tutored me in my fourth year at Oxford. He was a charming but laconic man with wry sense of humour as is often found in his profession. In one tutorial, we were discussing venereal disease. He quoted from the Bible, "The rain falls on the just and unjust alike." After a pause, he added with a smile, "but a bit more on the unjust!"

The tutorials were the core of the teaching. There were also lectures some mornings but no other formal teaching for the rest of the day. The dissecting room in the anatomy department was open from nine to five, Monday to Friday. Each cadaver was assigned to a group of four undergraduates, and the group was expected to complete the dissection of the whole body in five terms. Every two weeks, there was a formal viva to test anatomical knowledge on the part of the body we had just dissected, and every viva had to be passed. If you failed, then another date was set for a few days later, and back you went until that viva was passed.

A curious reader may wonder how the cadavers were so satisfactorily preserved. As soon after death as possible, the body donated for the teaching of anatomy was injected, under pressure, via a femoral artery with a large volume of formaldehyde. The formaldehyde circulates everywhere in the body, bathing all the tissues in the fluid and so preserving them. The only problem was the smell of formaldehyde, which stuck to one's hands and clothes and was difficult to wash off. We did not use gloves when we were dissecting. This was, after all, the early sixties, and hepatitis C, D, and HIV, were unknown. No dissector in those days caught any disease from these carefully preserved cadavers. At the completion of the dissection all the tissues, which were always carefully kept, would go for burial or cremation as laid down in the will of the person who had donated their body.

These dissections were a long time after the days of the body snatchers, of whom the famous John Hunter (1728-1793) was one. Hunter was without doubt a man of the Age of Enlightenment, when curiosity swept Western Europe. In anatomy and comparative anatomy, he was pre-eminent in the second half of the eighteenth century. He was the founder, in the eighteenth century, of modern surgery, a heroic figure who probably carried out more dissections than any other man. In 1754 he worked in his brother William's anatomy school in London and later in his own dissecting room in his house in Leicester Square.

As a result of the many cadaveric dissections he performed, he learned the anatomy of the human body in detail, and at the same time he taught new generations of surgeons. It is said that he introduced the idea of "principles" of surgery and rational explanations of repair and a scientic basis of operations. Some of the many specimins from his experiments survived the depredations of time and the bombing of the Second World War, and can be seen in the magnificent Hunterian Museum at the Royal College of Surgeons of England. Hunter also dissected many animals, both common and exotic, and made detailed comparisons between species. His prodigious output has benefitted science and surgery. The knowledge so gained was part of the background that led to the explosion of new operations that were first carried out a century later in the last decades of the nineteenth century. I am informed at the time of writing (2014) that the British medical schools have virtually abandoned dissection of cadavers, and medical students now spend relatively little time studying anatomy. This seems to represent a demotion for the foundation science of surgery.

There were lighter moments. To complete our anatomy studies early, in less than five terms, many undergraduates of my year spent several weeks of the 1963 summer vacation dissecting in the Anatomy Department of Bristol University who laid on the facilities for us.

Completion of our vacation dissection at Bristol freed up the fifth term at Oxford so we could concentrate on the first formal medical examination at the end of that term. This was the first part of the bachelor of medicine and surgery degree, which when passed, allowed medical students to start the clinical training. Following success in this examination, preparation was made to sit for the Bachelor of Arts degree (BA) in animal physiology at the end of the third year.

The time spent on the BA was made more interesting by study of human physiology in greater depth as well comparative physiology and embryology. Dr Torrence was my tutor, and I remember to this day his tutorials on the comparative physiology of respiration in different classes of animals in his rooms in St John's College.

This knowledge of comparative anatomy and physiology added interest when I was teaching medical students years later.

The understanding of genetics underwent a seminal advance in 1953 and blossomed by the end of the century. This advance was made alive for me in 1962, when I went to a lecture given by Dr Francis Crick[1], the co-discoverer of the double-helix structure of DNA, for which he was awarded the Nobel Prize in Medicine or Physiology. For anyone who has not done so, it is worth reading Watson and Crick's paper in *Nature* for its clarity and brevity. Dr Crick received a standing ovation for his lecture.

After being awarded a BA, with a second class degree in animal physiology, at the end of my third year, I stayed on at Oxford for a further two terms to study pathology and pharmacology and take examinations, which I passed. I then went down from Oxford in the summer of 1966 after a most enjoyable time.

---

[1] Watson, J.D. and Crick, F. H. C., A Structure for Deoxyribose Nucleic Acid, *Nature* 171 (1953): 737–738. Dr Crick's co-Nobel Laureates were James Watson and Maurice Wilkins.

CHAPTER 2

A Student at St Thomas's Hospital, London, 1966–1968

The clinical year was very different from the Oxford terms and was continuous, with no formal vacations. Each student could take two weeks' holiday a year. I lived throughout this time, at 19 Middleton Square in Islington with friends who were also medical students, except when on "take" at the hospital. The reason for this was that my parents were abroad during most of my student life. At this time, my father was a British-government-sponsored adviser to the ministry of agriculture in Emperor Haile Selassie's government in Ethiopia.

Each student was attached to a firm of physicians or surgeons for several months and during this time lived in the hospital whenever the firm was on take. There were four firms each for medicine and surgery at St Thomas's Hospital. A firm of surgeons and a firm of physicians were on call for all emergencies one week in four. During these "takes," the firm on duty was responsible for the admission and care of all emergency cases. The students attached to the firm on take were not allowed to leave the hospital without the permission of the dean, which was rarely granted. The surgical firm to which I was attached was that of Mr R. W. Nevin, who was dean of the medical school, and with him Mr H. E. Lockhart-Mummery, both general surgeons with a special interest in colorectal surgery. I will say more about my chiefs later.

The students were hands-on and learned to actually operate on lumps and bumps, drain abscesses, sew up wounds, and clerk emergency admissions. This latter necessitated taking a full history from each emergency admission followed by a detailed physical examination. We were expected to make a working diagnosis and start the initial treatment for the condition using this diagnosis, such as taking bloods for tests and putting up a drip if indicated. This was all checked by the house officer, who also clerked the patients. If an emergency operation was indicated, the registrar or senior registrar on call was informed and would take charge. Then there was an opportunity to assist at the operation, scrubbing up and holding a retractor for the surgeon, which gave a first-class view of all that was going on.

It is interesting to look back and remember that if there was difficulty putting up a drip, then it was the student's task, after training, to cut down onto and place a cannula in the long saphenous vein at the ankle. This technique of cutting down on to the vein, which I carried out on several occasions when patients were collapsed and shocked, had become common practice during the Second World War. However, it was usual to insert a plastic cannula straight into the vein and then tie it in place, rather than use the brass cannula still supplied in the hospital sterile packs for just such an occasion. I still have in my possession one of these metal cannulas[1].

If urgent operations were necessary at night, which occurred frequently, the students stayed up. Then after having breakfasted, the firm started with the normal tasks of the day at nine in the morning as usual. These included attending routine operating lists, ward rounds, outpatient clinics, lectures, and autopsies. Autopsies were carried out on all patients who died and had to be attended by

---

[1] Keynes, G. Editor. Blood Transfusion. John Wright and Sons, London, 1949.

the students. Seeing the direct visual evidence of the consequences of the disease process and resulting pathological changes that afflicted the patient when clerked on admission was a powerful way to learn.

No concessions were ever made or expected for loss of sleep, and I do not remember any mistakes made because of tiredness. Everything was checked by the houseman and registrar or senior registrar, so no student acted alone. There was also the advantage that during the night, it was possible to work with far fewer interruptions, it being quiet and dark, and the telephone rang only for emergencies. I continued to enjoy working through the night until I was in my late forties.

Acute appendicitis was common, and the clerk (student) who admitted and examined such a patient was expected to assist at the operation and even do a little operating under the direct supervision of the registrar. Perforated or bleeding ulcers were also common. Endoscopy did not exist, and both of these conditions, if severe, could only be treated by emergency surgery. Operating on a bleeding ulcer was often very difficult. Not only was the stomach full of blood, but also it was technically very difficult to gain access to the bleeding artery in the base of an ulcer on the posterior wall of the duodenum. The material used for under-running the spurting artery was catgut. Catgut was also used to close the duodenotomy made to gain access to the ulcer and to close the abdominal wall in layers. This suture material holds its full tensile strength for up to eighteen days before beginning to dissolve. However, if it weakened earlier, then complications were not uncommon. Rebleeding of a duodenal ulcer was particularly serious, as a second operation was even more difficult. In addition, the abdominal wounds gave way occasionally, causing a "burst abdomen," which also required another anaesthetic and a difficult resuturing. The surgeon had sometimes to close the abdominal wall against the contraction of the muscles, which were squeezing the bowels out through the incision under pressure.

Another very common emergency was acute obstruction of the bowel, often caused by adhesions following previous abdominal surgery or a colonic cancer. The adage used by older surgeons was: "Never allow the sun to rise or set on a case of obstruction," by which they meant that it was necessary to proceed to an operation as quickly as possible to give the patient with an obstruction the best chance of survival.

There are several reasons for this. The first is to restore a normal circulating fluid volume to maintain the blood pressure and perfusion of the vital organs. In bowel obstruction, the patient loses fluids in several ways. Vomiting is compounded by the continued secretion of saliva, gastric, pancreatic, and small-bowel juices. The bowel above the obstruction distends as the normal physiological absorption of fluid is inhibited, and as the normal secretions continue, they are effectively lost from the circulation, which in turn makes the patient's dehydration worse the longer the treatment is delayed. This distension sometimes results in rupture of the bowel, which is often fatal.

There is no doubt that in the sixties patients delayed coming to hospital and often presented as critically ill, and at the end stage of their obstruction. A nasogastric tube was passed to relieve the vomiting, and rapid rehydration was instituted to prepare them for surgery within a few hours of admission.

When on take, the duty firm would gather before nine on the Monday morning of the take week and not leave the hospital until the following Monday evening. This overlap meant that the new firm would take all admitted emergencies under their care from nine in the morning on Monday, while the firm ending their duty had the whole day to treat any urgent cases from the previous evening and then hand over any patient still needing surgery. The gain from this concentrated process was that the experience was unparalleled in width and depth, and students gained familiarity with many conditions. By attending the operations, I developed a taste for operating, which was augmented by the minor procedures I carried out in casualty, as the A&E departments were then known, all this while not missing out on the routine daytime clinical teaching.

The patients had round-the-clock care by the take firm, consisting of the senior registrar, registrar, and houseman, as well as formal twice-weekly consultant rounds. They were all seen and examined twice each day, including postoperatively, until discharged. This was indeed continuity of care.

Mr Brendan Devlin, one of the senior registrars, explained that there was a brief period in a surgeon's life when he could be "all things to all men." By this he meant that with the accumulation of practical experience and knowledge over a very broad front, the surgeon would have the knowledge, experience, and stamina to clerk, resuscitate, operate, and look after all his patients, both elective and emergency, round the clock as necessary. This is being "all things to all men." In the training period, experience and knowledge has yet to be gained, while stamina is there. As age advances, there is a great increase of experience but stamina declines. He also added that to be successful as a surgeon, it was necessary to have the three 'As'; ability, availability and affability.

The week on take did not mean that we got no sleep; most nights there would be several hours sleep, maybe broken by new emergencies coming in and needing clerking. Being "all things to all men" lasted, in my personal experience, from my late twenties into the late forties. By the latter age, the surgeon might well be able to work for twenty-four hours non-stop, but twenty-four hours later he would not be fit to operate without previously catching up on the lack of sleep.

Using the masculine gender only is not in any way disrespectful or avoiding recognition of the excellent women doctors and the very few women surgeons already established when I was training in the sixties and seventies. It is just a fact that I was not trained by a single consultant surgeon who was a woman throughout the twelve years of my postgraduate training before becoming a consultant. It should come as no surprise, that in the clinical student intake of my year, 1966, only 15% were women. This is how it was then; it has now changed.

The one notable exception, of a woman surgeon, was Miss Connie Fozzard[1], FRCOG, who was the senior registrar in obstetrics at the Central Middlesex Hospital when John Maddison and I, as students, were attached to the maternity unit to learn our obstetrics. Miss Fozzard was a good teacher. As an aside, we did all our deliveries at night, as the deliveries by day were taken by the student midwives!

Student days at St Thomas's were good.

[1]I met Miss Fozzard again in the eighties when she was a consultant obstretrician and gynaecologist and married to Dr Bunt White the haematologist at the RAEI in Wigan. If I was doing an interesting operation on a weekend they sometimes came to observe.

CHAPTER 3

"On the House" at St Thomas's Hospital, 1969

Following success in the finals and now entitled to be called Dr Maybury, I was privileged that Mr R. W. Nevin, dean of the medical school, appointed me as his house officer. There were, in fact, two housemen attached to the firm, and Patrick Wheeler and I alternated on night and weekend duties. Of course, we both worked through each weekday as normal. We considered ourselves lucky, as this was the first time that two house officers had been appointed to each firm. Before our appointment, a single houseman lived in as house surgeon—full time for the whole six months. In other words, day and night and every weekend, he had to be on hand to look after his chief's patients. In theory it was possible to have the odd weekend off, but in practice it was very difficult, as the incumbent had to find a substitute to look after the patients, and since the locum would not know the patients, continuity of care would be compromised. On these grounds alone, leave was thoroughly disapproved of by the chiefs, and consequently leave was never granted except for emergencies.

So Patrick Wheeler and I both worked every weekday and alternate nights by rotation as noted. As was accepted—and at that time never commented on—no concession was made for time worked at night, which happened quite frequently. Sometimes it was quiet, apart from the routine eleven o'clock ward round every night. During the firm's week on take, both house surgeons lived in for the whole week. We would often be up most of the night admitting and clerking patients after the students had carried out the preliminary examinations. We also initiated resuscitation of patients admitted as emergencies by the clerk (student) and assisted at operations. Even if one had worked through the night, the next day's work started at 8.00 a.m. with Mr Nevin's regular business ward round.

All house officers were given a charge, a printed sheet of instructions that included the statement that house officers were to "see all the patients charged to your care twice in every day," so we carried out a ward round, seeing and examining every patient in our care during the morning and late at night. If we found anything outside our competence, which at the beginning was just about everything, the house officer was to "refer the matter to his seniors and not meddle further therein." The language was beautiful.

Mr R W Nevin's firm consisted of two consultants as already noted: himself and Mr H. E. Lockhart-Mummery, who later became Serjeant Surgeon to HM the Queen and was knighted. Both chiefs were general surgeons, and both had a special interest in colorectal surgery. The senior registrar was Mr Brendon Devlin, the registrar was Mr Terry Brightmore, and the most junior were the house officers, Patrick Wheeler and me. It is of interest to note that there were no senior house officers. A progression of promotion through the surgical grades at St Thomas's was not possible, as all aspiring surgeons had to leave the alma mater to gain experience elsewhere and take and pass the examination to become fellows of the Royal College of Surgeons (FRCS) before being eligible to apply for a registrar's post at St Thomas's or elsewhere.

During the week, Mr Nevin lived in a flat in Lambeth Palace just a short walk from the hospital and at weekends went home to the country. It was his habit to come into the hospital every day at eight o'clock to be met at the front entrance by the house surgeon, who had been on duty the night before, to conduct a round of all his patients. This was a business round, and there were never students present. Mr Nevin's patients were nursed on two wards but could be scattered elsewhere in the hospital, depending on bed availability. We went methodically from ward to ward and were joined by the sister of each ward as we entered. All the patients were very well known to me, because I'd clerked them on their admission, assisted at any operation they underwent, and also, as a matter of course, reviewed them twice a day on house officer rounds. With Mr Nevin in the morning—apart from new patients, either elective or emergencies—no time was wasted presenting a history, for they were well known to him. He always greeted each patient cheerfully and by name and enquired of me about their well-being. If the reply was, "Everything is fine, sir" or similar, and the ward sister nodded in agreement, we moved on to the next patient.

All patients for an operation that day would be examined by Mr Nevin to check the diagnosis and be sure the operation was still in the patient's best interest. Then if it was a question of the left or the right side to be operated on, the relevant side of the patient was marked with an indelible pen to ensure there were no mistakes made.

Postoperative patients who were unwell were carefully examined, and instructions were given by the chief for their care. On the rare occasions that a further operation was needed, there was time for it to be arranged later that day after any necessary tests had been carried out, which the house officer organised immediately. I learned a great deal from Mr Nevin, not only from his extensive knowledge and experience but also about how to treat people in a polite and civilised fashion. At nine o'clock we went about our routine daily duties, knowing that everyone had been seen on the wards, and anything that needed doing had been done or could be arranged. Mr Nevin never appeared hurried. However, if a member of his staff did something crass, he could be very angry. It was an awesome sight. It only happened twice while I was working for him, and I am glad to say that on neither occasion was it directed at me.

Today it may well seem strange that so much operating went on during the night, as by the end of the twentieth century operations at night were generally only allowed for uncontrolled haemorrhage. Most patients with a serious abdominal condition now spend the night being resuscitated before an operation. Fluid or blood losses are replaced, and the blood pressure is stabilised, thus protecting renal function. Also, in cases of infection, antibiotic treatment is started. In present times, such a patient is then operated on in a dedicated emergency operating theatre during the day, ideally with a consultant anaesthetist and a consultant surgeon present.

The common emergencies in the late sixties were obstructions, including perforations, diverticulitis with perforation or associated abscess, obstructed hernias, acute appendicitis, prostatic hyperplasia causing acute or chronic retention of urine, and significant intestinal bleeding due to gastric or duodenal ulcers. This, of course, meant operating during the evening and night. Endoscopy, CT, or MRI scanners were still in the future. This policy was right at that time and saved many a patient. It was also a very efficient way to use the operating theatres and was very cheap, as doctors were not paid any overtime for night and weekend duties. This was just how it was at that time, and I cannot remember the subject ever being discussed. It was, after all, only a couple of years earlier that housemen were not paid at all! However, the volume and constancy of the work meant that a young aspiring surgeon like me learned and saw a phenomenal amount in a short time, as we were always in the hospital and always on duty. It was a true apprenticeship, and I thrived on it.

House Physician at Wexham Park Hospital, Slough

Wexham Park Hospital was new, and its architecture won prizes. The hospital consisted of a central tower seven stories high, with arms of a single story radiating out like a star from the base of the tower. These contained the wards and casualty. It was one of the first hospitals to have a helicopter landing pad; there was an interesting episode concerning a helicopter that I will describe later. The doctors' mess was on the sixth floor of the tower block and the doctors' residence on the seventh, a splendid place with huge plate-glass windows and panoramic views.

When a cardiac arrest occurred, speed to reach the relevant ward from the mess was very important. By the time I reached the ward, the staff nurse had already brought the cardiac arrest trolley to the patient's bedside and drawn the curtains around. Calls from casualty were responded to in the same way. On one occasion, I arrived to find a patient who had a bowel obstruction was cyanosed, because she had already aspirated gastric fluid into her trachea, which caused breathing difficulties. I immediately slipped an endotracheal tube into her trachea. I just had time to blow up the balloon to prevent any further fluid from entering the lungs when she vomited a large quantity of fluid. Without this intervention, a further aspiration of gastric fluid would certainly have killed her. The bronchi were then washed out with saline, and an intravenous drip and nasogastric tube were inserted before I handed the patient over to the surgical team, who operated later that night. The lady survived. Results like these were always very pleasing.

I enjoyed my time at Wexham Park Hospital and learned a great deal of medicine during my six-month stay. Dr Prakash, the medical registrar on my firm, was Burmese of Indian origin and had escaped from the military dictatorship. He was an amiable and patient man who went out of his way to teach me. Within only a few weeks under his close supervision, I was managing the admission and initial treatment of patients with diabetic precoma, myocardial infarctions, and gastro-intestinal emergencies. Dr Prakash was always at the end of the phone, and I always kept him informed of what was happening. He often came down from the mess to see that everything was as it should be. Funnily enough, I preferred the work as a house physician to that of a house surgeon. My reasons were in no way disrespectful to my excellent chiefs at St Thomas's. It was simply that in medicine I was able to immediately initiate definitive treatment of the patients admitted, if it was within my experience to do so. In surgery, although the house surgeon would clerk patients and put up drips, etc., the registrar always had to be called, and it was he who would take the decision whether to operate or not on the patient in question.

Dr Peter Reed, an extremely knowledgeable consultant physician, was one of my chiefs. I learned a great deal of theoretical medicine during his post-take ward rounds, which were always conducted with the notes in sister's office with occasional forays into the ward. There were frequently patients with liver failure on the ward. One very jaundiced young man was of particular concern to Dr Reed. After reviewing the patient, he rang Professor Sheila Sherlock at the Royal Free Hospital. At the end of this conversation, Dr Reed turned to me and told me that the professor had asked for the patient to be transferred to the Royal Free as fast as possible. Please would I arrange it? Being naive and taking Dr Reed at his word, I rang the RAF and arranged a helicopter transfer within the hour. The patient was duly delivered, and all seemed well until the bill arrived on the hospital secretary's desk. It was several hundred pounds—a considerable sum. I was then summoned by Dr Reed, and I told him what I had done. He just nodded and added that I should speak to him before arranging helicopter transfer in the future. I heard nothing more.

My other chief was Dr Gerald Thomas, a consultant cardiologist, himself trained by the great Dr Wood of *"Wood's Cardiology."* Dr Thomas told me that when Dr Wood himself developed chest pain, he did not recognise its cause, although he was, in fact, having an infarct. Dr Thomas's style of ward round was to reach the first bed and after introduction to his patient ask me what was going on. On my first round, I started with the history and presentation at full length. I could see he was becoming increasingly impatient, and finally he stopped me and asked if the patient was all right. I replied in the affirmative, and he immediately moved on to the next bed. If the previous night's take had been light, with no patients with difficult problems, then the round was very short, and we decamped to sister's office for coffee. Dr Thomas, of course, knew that Dr Prakash and I had already been round to review everybody before he had arrived.

However, if my response to his usual question was that there was a problem or difficulty in diagnosis, his whole demeanour changed, and he became totally focused on that patient. I then presented a succinct history, and after he had asked further questions of the patient, he would carry out a detailed examination, teaching as he went. This was followed by reading the ECG and evaluating any other tests available. Much discussion followed to develop a working diagnosis and a plan of action. Dr Thomas taught me a great deal, and even years later when I was a consultant surgeon, I still carried a stethoscope and used it daily. Perhaps I was the only consultant general surgeon to routinely carry a stethoscope and read ECGs.

CHAPTER 4:

Casualty Officer and Prosector of Anatomy

The first professional surgical examination that had to be negotiated was the primary FRCS, which required the completion of two house jobs and six months in a post as casualty officer (A&E SHO) before taking the examination. When I was working for him, Mr Nevin had advised me to apply for a casualty post at St Thomas's that would last for six months. It would be followed automatically, if my application was successful, with a similar period as prosector in the department of anatomy of the medical school. I applied and was very glad to have been successful. Casualty was great fun and was also the only training post in those days that was worked in shifts, being the only job that did not need continuity of care, as all the patients were either sent home or admitted under the relevant speciality.

There was a great variety of work ranging from dealing with cuts and abrasions, draining abscesses, and setting fractures to performing cardiac resuscitation and resuscitation of traffic accident victims, to mention a few of the tasks we undertook. The casualty officers (COs) examined all patients who came into casualty, making the initial working diagnosis and carrying out treatment in minor cases. With emergencies, the CO initiated resuscitation immediately while calling for assistance from a more senior colleague, or in serious cases he called the resident surgical officer (RSO) or resident medical officer (RMO) as appropriate.

The RSO and RMO were at the very pinnacle of the training ladder. These posts lasted two years, and their conditions of employment stipulated that the RSO and RMO were resident. They literally lived in the hospital for the whole two years. They were very well looked after, each with a splendid suite of rooms, meals, and everything domestic done for them. Most RSOs left at the end of their contract having been appointed as consultants to the most prestigious jobs.

There was one major drawback,—hearsay had it that all those who were married before they accepted the post were divorced during their tenure. These appointments must have been the last jobs in a twentieth-century democracy where there was absolutely no allowance at all for any life outside work. However, when they finished the two-year contract, the former RSOs and RMOs were truly masters of surgery or medicine, having accumulated unparalleled experience during their tenure. The RSO would have carried out operations on the total range of surgical procedures then part of the general surgical repertoire, as all the major emergency surgery at night was carried out by the RSO. Living in all the time meant they knew everything that was going on in the hospital. Also, they spent a lot of time teaching.

Rumour then had it that the next group of senior registrars, from amongst whom the new RSO would be selected, decided amongst themselves that none would apply for the post. They carried out their threat, and the posts of RSO and RMO lapsed. From then on, the senior registrar of each of the four firms would live in for their week on take.

Late one night, while I was having a coffee break in the nurse's station at the front of casualty, we heard the most terrible banging on the glass front of the building. A man of about twenty was running along, hammering on the glass screaming, "I'm dying! Let me in! I'm dying! Let me in!" We were used to drunks and other rowdy elements, but this did not seem to me to be quite the case, and so I went out to meet him.

He was quite incoherent and distressed, so I took him straight to the resuscitation room and laid him on one of the couches. I could not feel a pulse, so I immediately attached him to an ECG, which showed his heart was beating at just under 200 beats a minute with long runs of ventricular ectopic beats. This is a sure sign that a cardiac arrest may occur at any moment due to the disorganisation of nerve conduction in the heart. I could get no sense out of the patient, and as soon as I saw the ECG, I put a drip up to give venous access for drugs and infused lignocaine to calm the heart. Gradually the ectopic beats became less threatening, and the young man began to recover.

Apparently he had been at his girlfriend's flat, and after a drink she had offered him some cake, of which he had eaten two generous slices. Almost immediately he felt very ill, with the sensation that he was about to die. The place he came from was only a few hundred yards away from casualty, and he came running. His girlfriend, who turned up later, admitted that she had baked a substantial quantity of cannabis into the cake. She had not got round to eating a piece herself due to all the commotion. The man came to no harm and was discharged the next morning from the observation ward. Thus I was introduced to the effects of cannabis and the acute dangers it can pose when cooked and eaten. It is obviously not denatured by baking!

Another more salutary experience was one afternoon when the call came in that an attempted suicide had jumped off a footbridge over the Waterloo Road. After she hit the road, she had been struck by a passing car. Another CO and I started resuscitation. She was conscious but totally uncooperative and in a very bad way, with three limbs broken, a major abdominal injury, and a head injury.

We were about to intubate her to secure her respiration when she pulled herself together just long enough to curse us for interfering fools—but in rather more explicit terms. We did intubate her, but she died a few minutes later of her injuries. She had intended her suicide attempt to be successful and did not want to be thwarted by interfering doctors. She succeeded in spite of our best endeavours.

The casualty officers also had more routine work. St Thomas's at that time offered a same-day second opinion to local GPs for patients who had developed acute back pain. This condition, if severe, can be very disabling. The Department of Physical Medicine was headed by Dr James Cyriax[1], a great protagonist of same-day manipulation for patients with acute back pain. Patients suffering from this condition were sent by their general practitioner to St Thomas's casualty with a handwritten note and seen by one of the COs, who took a detailed history and performed a physical examination, which included an internal examination in men to exclude cancer of the prostate. A plain X-ray of the back was carried out and checked by the CO. If there were no abnormalities, the patients were sent straightaway to the Department of Physical Medicine and had their backs manipulated the same day. All these patients were given a three-week follow-up appointment for review by the same casualty officer they had first seen.

This example of continuity of care meant we could see for ourselves the effect of the manipulation, and the result was recorded. These results were most interesting and showed that 30% of these patients with severe acute-onset back pain were cured after one manipulation by Dr Cyriax. Those who still had severe pain were referred for a second manipulation the day of review, and about a third of these responded and could return to work. On several occasions, if casualty was quiet, I would accompany the patients and watch Dr Cyriax[1] manipulate their backs, which was a very

---

[1] Cyriax, J. Textbook of Orthopaedic medicine, Vol. 1. Diagnosis of soft tissue lesions, 4th Ed. Cassell, London, 1962.

physical and skilled procedure. I was most impressed and could never understand why the technique did not become widely used by the NHS.

Casualty was an interesting six months of very practical medicine. There was always someone more senior around to advise, help, or demonstrate what to do. We learned in emergency situations to resuscitate logically and intubate safely, place chest and abdominal drains, and many other techniques and also frequently went to theatre to assist the RSO with his operations. Emergency surgery has a great advantage over most other branches of medicine in that, having made a diagnosis following the clerking of the patient, the preoperative diagnosis was rapidly proved correct or not at the operation. This provided instant feedback that honed one's skill and confidence in making a diagnosis that could then be applied to future cases. At that time (1970) the diagnosis was always clinical, made from history, when available, and careful and logical examination. Apart from plain X-rays, there were no other preoperative means of visualising the internal effects of injuries or diseases.

Prosector of Anatomy

At the end of the casualty job, I moved over to the anatomy department in the preclinical part of the medical school. Next to the brightly lit dissecting room where the cadavers were laid out was a small room with a table that I shared with Ian Reynolds, John Black, and John Dove. Nearly forty years later, John Black became the president of the Royal College of Surgeons. Back in our office we were next door to Professor Davies, editor of the latest edition of *Gray's Anatomy*, which was to be our bible for the next six months. We taught the students over the dissections, also received regular tutorials, and had many discussions about anatomy over coffee. It was an exceedingly pleasant time. Towards the end of the six months, we all passed the primary fellowship examination. Now we were all ready to develop our careers in surgery. I have always been grateful for this thorough grounding in anatomy, especially later when dealing with complex operations; this very detailed knowledge of anatomy served me well.

It was apparent to the prosectors that there had been a significant change in the approach to teaching since we had been up at university only a few years before. The students we were teaching were going through their preclinical training at St Thomas's Hospital Medical School having come straight from school. Their working week was completely organised from nine in the morning to five in the evening every day except the weekend. This rigorous programme, where a student's presence must be accounted for at all times, left no time for serious outside activities such as sport. It is impossible to play any sport seriously when only practicing at the weekends. The prosectors remonstrated with Professor Davis on behalf of the students without success. We were only suggesting that the curriculum be cut back on Wednesday to allow the afternoon for other activities, but again to no avail.

With the knowledge I'd gained so far, I was now ready to learn the science and art of the practice of surgery in earnest.

CHAPTER 5

Surgical Registrar at Warwick Hospital, 1971–1973

Warwick Hospital was part of a group of hospitals that also included Leamington Spa and Stratford Hospitals. They were served by three consultant general surgeons: Mr Christopher Savage, a general and vascular surgeon based at Leamington Spa, who had one list a week for vascular operations at Warwick Hospital; Mr Michael Lord at Stratford-upon-Avon Hospital; and Mr John Marsh at Warwick Hospital. Mr Marsh had interviewed me and appointed me as his registrar to be based at Warwick, with which I was delighted.

Mr Marsh ran the surgical firm at Warwick Hospital. Mr Savage visited once a week. The junior staff included the registrar and two house officers. The surgical wards were named Ryland's and Clare Wards. A two-bed bay was being carved out of one of the wards to become the hospital's first intensive care unit, a fairly new concept that was now spreading to district general hospitals. The one and only casualty department for the whole hospital group was at Warwick and so was in my patch.

I underwent a baptism of fire. On arrival in Warwick, I was very inexperienced at operating, and Mr Marsh worked day and night to teach and supervise me. Within a few weeks I was doing all the emergency appendicectomies, strangulated hernias, and gastric or duodenal perforations, calling for Mr Marsh's advice or help whenever I was perplexed or worried, which was often in those first weeks. But as my confidence grew and my skill developed, the frequency with which I called in my chief tailed off. There was a golden rule: it was mandatory to call the chief early for advice or help when encountering something not dealt with before or that was proving difficult. By strict adherence to this rule, there were no disasters. As I made progress, Mr Marsh's confidence in me grew, so he allowed me to do more and more complex procedures. This was a most exciting time.

My work rota was awesome. In week one I was on duty every day and night, including the weekend, except for Wednesday afternoon and night. In the second week my duty rota was from Monday to Thursday day and night and also all day Friday. Friday night and the weekend I was off duty. Usually I could get away at six or seven on Friday evening. This two week rotation was then repeated. It amounted to being on call one hundred and fifty hours in the first week of the rota and one hundred and thirty seven hours the second week. This was a baptism of fire, but I enjoyed it enormously as under Mr Marsh's careful tutelage I made rapid progress. I did not mind the hours as I was accumulating experience at a tremendous pace having arrived at Warwick with very little experience of operating. The work was all absorbing and very busy all the time both day and night.

Every morning at eight, I carried out a full ward round with the two house officers and saw all the general surgical patients in the hospital. Any new patients admitted during the night would have already been brought to my attention, either by phone or, if more serious, by my coming in to see them. Those patients whom I was called in to see, and who needed an operation, were operated on during the night; if it was beyond my experience, Mr Marsh was informed, and he would come in to operate.

This was the era before seatbelts, and there were many car accidents with horrific injuries, including head injuries. Within a few weeks of my starting the job, Mr Marsh had taught me to clinically diagnose intracranial bleeding and to correctly place six burr holes in the skull to release pressure within the skull caused by haemorrhage. He also showed me how to raise a cranial (bone) flap to treat widespread subdural bleeding, and how to elevate depressed fractures of the skull. A visiting facio-maxillary surgeon came next day and operated on any malar, orbital (facial), or mandibular fractures admitted during the night.

Abdominal trauma was common, and Mr Marsh taught me to do emergency laparotomies and splenectomies. In the early seventies, a ruptured spleen was always removed entirely. All such patients needed subsequently to be vaccinated against pneumococcal infections and to take a daily dose of penicillin for life, because their resistance to some infections was compromised in the absence of the spleen.

I also learned to operate on bowel obstructions, which were frequent due to cancer of the colon, and always presented late in the natural history of the disease. The operation of choice at that time for these obstructed patients was to perform a colostomy above the level of the obstruction, so relieving the pressure in the bowel before it had built up to such a degree that the bowel ruptured. This procedure had a high success rate and enabled the patient to recover from the obstruction. A few weeks later, a definitive operation to excise the tumour and rejoin the bowel was performed, and the colostomy was closed. Sometimes this latter procedure was done at a third operation if considered safer for the patient.

Obstruction of the small bowel was also common and usually due to adhesions. It was caused by one or more loops of small bowel adhering to adjacent loops, so preventing the normal smooth sliding movement of one loop of bowel over another. This immobility can result in the bowel kinking and stopping the flow of the small-bowel contents, resulting in dilatation of the bowel above the kink as it filled with the normal secretions. In this situation,

Mr Marsh taught me the careful dissection technique needed to divide the adhesions without perforating the bowel. Adhesions were the commonest cause of bowel obstruction in the seventies. It was then discovered that the adhesions were often caused by an intense reaction of the peritoneum to chalk. Chalk was being used as a lubricant on surgical gloves to enable surgeons to pull them on with ease. The use of chalk as a lubricant was then stopped and the incidence of this cause of obstruction rapidly declined. This was a serious example of iatrogenic (doctor- or treatment-caused) disease.

I also assisted Mr Marsh at four routine operating lists a week, when I was allowed, under his direct supervision, to carry out part of the various operations he was performing. Once a week he had twin lists, with two theatres operating in parallel. I operated in one theatre, and Mr Marsh was next door. Initially only minor cases were placed on my list, but as I was learning fast, Mr Marsh added operations of increasing complexity.

Within a few months, I was able to carry out such operations as an uncomplicated right hemicolectomy and Millin's prostatectomy[1]. This latter operation was the old-fashioned open prostatectomy through a suprapubic abdominal incision. Millin's operation was hailed as a triumph when introduced in the forties and resulted in the mortality rate being reduced by 90%. This operation had been taught to Mr Marsh by Mr Millin himself. For this operation, I learned to use Millin's fearsome boomerang needle.

The boomerang needle he devised was very useful, but as mentioned, a fearsome instrument. It was used to close the prostatic capsule quickly and so reduce bleeding. Mr Marsh also told me that Millin operated without gloves, which was not uncommon at that time, but what was unusual is that he apparently deliberately allowed his right index fingernail to grow long so he could "winkle"

---

[1] Millin, T. Retropubic prostatectomy. Lancet 1945:249,693-6.

the prostate out using the nail to rapidly open the tissue plane between the capsule and the prostate itself.

One day in the middle of carrying out a Millin's prostatectomy, a problem arose, and a message was sent to the next theatre to ask for Mr Marsh's help. He was obviously very busy and said to the nurse who had brought the message, "Let him sweat a bit." He then came through a few minutes later and demonstrated how to deal with the problem.

To be a competent surgeon it was, and still is, essential to be assisting a chief when major technical problems arise. The apprentice then learns what can be and should be done in these circumstances. This knowledge cannot be acquired quickly. It requires long hours of operating and assisting to master the handling of such problems safely. The apprentice also learns what cannot be done and then understands the limitations of his or her craft. This way I learned many techniques from Mr Marsh that I used throughout my career.

By the end of my first year, Mr Marsh had taught me most of the operations he regularly carried out. Amongst them were abdomino-perineal excisions of the rectum, where he and I alternated being the abdominal and the perineal surgeon. Also solo, I had advanced to carrying out Billroth I and II gastrectomies for stomach cancers, gastric ulcers, and colectomies of all types. Mr Marsh taught me to do cholecystectomies and, where indicated, explorations of the common bile duct. On every operating list there was a patient with a chronic duodenal ulcer for vagotomy and pyloroplasty and a patient for haemorrhoidectomy.

Another field where I gained a lot of experience and learned to operate was on newborn babies with spina bifida (meningomyelocoele). The defect where the terminal part of the spinal cord is exposed was closed at operation to prevent continuous leakage of cerebro-spinal fluid (CSF). Then later, if a baby developed abnormally high intracranial pressure, I learned to insert a Spitz-Holter valve to prevent hydrocephalus. This was an interesting technique where one end of a tube was inserted into a cerebral ventricle. The other end was inserted into the jugular vein or placed into the peritoneal cavity. The tube between was tunnelled subcutaneously. In the middle of the tube was a one-way valve that could be gently pumped to restore flow if it was blocked.

From Mr Savage, I learned the technique of harvesting arteries from cadavers and assisted him when he operated using these homografts to replace diseased and obstructed vessels. While I was working at Warwick, commercially manufactured synthetic grafts became available for the first time, so the harvesting of vessels from cadavers was no longer needed and became an obsolete skill

Historically, in World War I, wounded men rarely arrived at an equipped hospital in less than thirteen days. This time lag was halved in World War II. However, vascular injuries need to be operated on quickly for success in saving tissues beyond the injury. This was first accomplished—often within an hour of infliction of the wound—during the Korean War (1950–1953). This was the first time helicopters were used routinely to lift casualties from the battle zone and deliver them directly to a mobile army surgical hospital (MASH). Many will remember an exciting American television series of the same name illustrating the benefit of helicopter transport for the wounded, among other things! Some progress was made in Korea to successfully reduce the number of amputations following wounds to peripheral arteries. However the greatest advances in treatment were achieved in the Vietnam War between 1955 and the fall of Saigon in 1975, when the wounded were delivered often in minutes to a fully equipped MASH.

War was thus the crucible for the development of vascular surgery, which was a mid-twentieth-century revolution in treatment. One of the great pioneers was Michael E. DeBakey, whose work led to use of the MASHs behind the battle zone. Then, during the Vietnam War his work led to the production of synthetic grafts.

With modern anaesthetics (including muscle relaxants), simple intravenous techniques, and the availability of synthetic grafts, it was possible not only to repair but replace badly damaged or shot-away arteries.

More prosaically, new anaesthetic techniques spread quickly and were used in Warwick Hospital. Once a week I did a list of minor operations with Dr Larade, the senior consultant anaesthetist. The list would usually consist of ten to twelve patients in a half-day operating session of four hours. This huge throughput was possible due to the skill and expertise of Dr Larade, who had three patients asleep simultaneously: one in the anaesthetic room being anaesthetised, one being operated on, and one in the recovery room, waking up. He had one nurse as an assistant. There were never any problems with patient safety while I was working at Warwick. Meanwhile, Sister Sullivan, the theatre sister, had the instruments for every procedure ready on separate trolleys. The moment I had finished one operation and the patient was taken to the recovery room, the next patient was brought in and placed on the operating table. Sister Sullivan took the "dirty" trolley out, scrubbed and gowned for the next procedure, and placed the new trolley with sterile instruments ready. I just had time to write the operation notes and scrub before immediately starting operating on the next patient. During those early months as a very junior surgeon, I had only to hold out my hand and Sister Sullivan invariably gave me the correct instrument, simultaneously telling me the name of the instrument. The result was that I knew the names of all the instruments within weeks.

The emergencies that poured into Warwick Hospital's casualty included many road traffic accidents. At that time no one had evaluated the risk of drink-driving, and people thought that there was no reason not to drive just because you had had a few drinks at a pub. It was only slowly realised in accident and emergency departments, such as Warwick, just how many accidents were due to drink-driving. People, always men, drove far too fast along narrow and dangerous roads with a high blood-alcohol level, so it is not surprising that there were so many accidents and so many injuries.

In the early seventies, Warwick Hospital took in a major traffic accident about every ten days. Usually there were several seriously injured casualties. It was at this time that lobbying for compulsory seat belts was gathering momentum, and Warwick Hospital took part in a survey of all road traffic accidents admitted. In a short time, it was easy to identify the pattern of injuries, depending on the type of vehicle and where the injured had been sitting in the vehicle. This research programme was run by the then-Birmingham Accident Hospital to which we sent our records and observations.

As a result of these observations, all general surgeons of that time have engraved on their minds the pattern of injuries caused by road traffic accidents (RTAs). When a car halts abruptly in an accident, the driver continues moving forward at the speed of the car before impact. His chest hit the centre of the steering wheel, often fracturing the ribs on either side of the sternum, which causes a flail chest. When attempting to take the next breath, the sternum collapses inwards with little or no air entering the lungs. Without oxygen, that person's life is in imminent peril, and urgent intubation of the trachea becomes mandatory. Without artificial ventilation, to restore the oxygenation of the blood, death was inevitable for many of these patients. So the small intensive care unit at Warwick Hospital was put to excellent use looking after these patients.

The driver would receive further horrific injuries as his head continued to move forwards, often catching his chin on the upper rim of the steering wheel and fracturing the jaw. The head would keep moving over the steering wheel and crash into the windscreen, smashing it, which resulted in terrible scalp and facial lacerations from the broken glass. The scalp wounds alone could result in considerable blood loss, and the facial lacerations resulted in appalling disfigurement. The shoulders would move forwards and up, often fracturing the humeri and the collar-bones. The abdomen would often be rammed into the lower rim of the steering wheel, and intra-abdominal injuries included rupture of the spleen or the liver. The steering wheels of the seventies were much larger than those in modern cars, because more leverage was needed, as there was no power steering. Meanwhile the legs were also moving forward at speed. The knees hit the dashboard, causing either dislocation or fracture of one or both hips or femurs. The lower legs swung forwards hitting the dashboard fascia, inflicting fractures of the tibias and fibulas of one or both legs.

The front-seat passenger would not get the flail chest or fractured mandible but could have even more severe lacerations of the scalp and face from smashing the windscreen. Injuries to the femurs and lower legs were similar to the driver's, and sometimes internal injuries also occurred.

The back-seat passengers could compound the injuries of those sitting in front by crashing into the seat in front, so propelling it forwards faster and farther than would otherwise have happened. The back-seat passenger's injuries could be horrendous but were usually of a lesser degree than were received by those in front. The results from Warwick helped add weight to the need for the compulsory fitting of seat belts.

Owners of cars registered in Britain on or after 1 January 1965 had been required by a law that came into effect on 31 December 1968 to have seat belts fitted in the front seats. Subsequently the requirement was extended to the back seats. The law mandating the compulsory wearing of seat belts for front-seat occupants, in the United Kingdom, only came into effect on 31 January 1983. Evidential breath testing was introduced at the same time. Seat belts are a proven way of reducing the severity of injuries. The government has estimated that since wearing seat belts was made compulsory in 1983, it has reduced casualties by at least 370 deaths and 7000 serious injuries per year for front-seat passengers and 70 deaths and 1,000 serious injuries for rear-seat passengers (DETR 1997).

It was unsurprising that the people involved in these accidents in the seventies were often dead on arrival in casualty. However, many survived, and they needed emergency resuscitation and surgery. The management of the injured was decided after careful clinical examination by a general surgeon who carried out or directed the treatment of these serious injuries. Apart from blood analysis and cross-matching, the only investigation available was the plain X-ray. There were no scanners, ultrasound, or endoscopes.

If there was breathing difficulty caused by a tension pneumothorax or flail chest, this was immediately treated appropriately in casualty. The cardiovascular status of the injured was assessed, and an intravenous cannula was inserted into a vein to take blood for analysis and cross-matching and to enable the infusion of appropriate fluids to stabilise the patient's blood pressure and replace blood lost in the accident. Careful note was taken of any head injury. If the injured person was unconscious on arrival in casualty, it was necessary to find out if he or she had responded or talked after the accident for even for a short time. This could be gleaned from the ambulance men and would indicate whether the brain was functioning after the accident. Subsequent loss of consciousness was probably due to a rise in intracranial pressure due to haemorrhage or oedema.

All bones were checked clinically for fractures, not forgetting the pelvis. A catheter was passed to assess and monitor urine output and thus renal function. An experienced team does not take long to make this initial assessment, and the speed with which the patient must be moved to theatre was dictated by the presence or absence of haemorrhage, intracranial or elsewhere. Every week or two I found myself operating—quite often simultaneously with an orthopaedic colleague—on the victims of major traffic trauma.

If subdural or extradural haemorrhage was suspected, then burr holes were indicated, and three were drilled on each side of the skull. There were many successes in relieving intracranial pressure from subdural and occasionally extradural haemorrhage with burr holes. Unhappily, and not infrequently, patients had gross oedema of the brain and very high intracranial pressure that was beyond treatment. From the clinical examination alone, it was not possible to reasonably decide whether such a patient was beyond salvage and therefore avoid an operation that would not achieve anything useful. So unless the patient had fixed, dilated pupils, they were operated on. In the unfortunate circumstances noted above, usually only one burr hole was needed to confirm that the patient was unsalvageable, as extrusion of brain due to the high intracranial pressure was immediately recognised by the surgeon. If it could be known in advance that a head injury was so severe that the patient would not survive, this knowledge would enable the surgical attendants to make them comfortable and avoid an operation. Several years later such a test became available. However, in the early seventies, the aggressive policy of operating when intracranial or intra-abdominal bleeding was suspected on clinical grounds meant that those with salvageable conditions were not missed and so not denied effective treatment.

Late one evening, I was phoned from casualty and told that one of our own consultants, a consultant gynaecologist, had been brought in following an accident. I was there in a flash and was met with an irremediable problem. He had crashed his open topped sports car into the back of a lorry, and the car had gone under the lorry's overhang behind the back wheels. He had taken a severe blow to the top of his head, which hit the tailboard of the lorry, partially decapitating him. I rang my chief and also the duty consultant neurosurgeon at the Birmingham Accident Hospital, but there was nothing to be done, and he was declared dead.

This injury has rarely been seen since. The overhang at the back of a lorry is a thing of the past. All lorries are now fitted with an impact-absorbing rear barrier that comes flush with the back of the lorry and reaches down so low that a car cannot get underneath. Professor Tisane at the Birmingham Accident Hospital published a paper in 1973, saying that the traffic characteristics of cars and lorries were largely incompatible and increased the likelihood of collisions and of extremely severe injuries to car occupants. "Some reduction in deaths may be expected from making lorries more conspicuous and eliminating the rear overhangs." He went on to say, less helpfully, "More fundamental measures are segregation of lorries from cars and return of heavy traffic to the railway." An overhang at the rear of a lorry is now a thing of the past.

There were many other emergencies. One night I was rung from Ryland's Ward and told that an RTA casualty with a fractured mandible was having difficulties breathing and was becoming cyanosed (blue) due to lack of oxygen. This man had crashed his car into a tree in an attempt to commit suicide and had been admitted from casualty for observation and to await the facio-maxillary surgeon's ward round the following day. In the meantime, oedema was causing obstruction of his airway. I asked the staff nurse to get an emergency tracheotomy pack from theatre immediately. Then I leapt into my trousers over my pyjamas, as it was late. Pulling on my white coat and shoes, I ran to the ward.

I was there within a minute and not a second too soon, as the man was deep purple and losing consciousness; his breathing was completely obstructed. There was no time to scrub or use local anaesthetic, as I could see he was about to have a cardiac arrest. The tracheotomy pack was already opened by the well-trained and efficient nurse. I immediately picked up the scalpel and made a vertical incision in his lower neck, cutting through the skin and the thyroid isthmus and into the trachea in one movement. Because he was close to cardiac arrest, there was virtually no bleeding. With a spreader, an instrument rather like a reverse forceps that opened its jaws on closure of the handle, the trachea was opened, and a hiss of air entered his lungs. I just had time to slip a tracheotomy tube into the opening and secure it, while the patient recovered consciousness. I went home feeling elated with the work done. The patient had his jaw plated by the facio-maxillary surgeon the next morning, and the swelling of his throat gradually settled over the next few days. He did not develop a wound infection, in spite of the lack of time to use aseptic procedures.

On another night I was called by the duty psychiatrist at the local asylum, as they were called at that time, which was a massive Victorian-built mental hospital in the country several miles from Warwick. It was an imposing brick building with turrets, set in several hundred acres of land. Patients who were fit and able worked on the land and produced most of the food for the hospital, which had a population of about a thousand patients and several hundred staff. Surplus produce could be sold. That night I was taken through door after door, each of which had to be unlocked and then locked behind me by the male nurse who accompanied me. We walked along lengthy corridors and finally came to the sanatorium, where the patient was in bed.

She was a middle-aged woman with an enormously distended abdomen and signs of peritonitis. I arranged for her to be transferred to Warwick Hospital immediately and returned to organise the preparations for surgery, as it was well after midnight. At operation, the colon was grossly thickened, indicating that the obstruction was of long standing, with massive distension and a small perforation in the lower abdomen caused by cancer of the sigmoid colon. The colonic cancer was resected, the upper end of the bowel was brought out onto the abdominal wall as a colostomy, and the upper end of the transected rectum was closed with sutures (Hartmann's procedure). A few hours later, when I was doing my daily ward round at eight in the morning, I came to the end of the bed occupied by this woman. To my surprise she was sitting up in bed and eating a cooked breakfast. A cooked breakfast was available for all patients in those days. "This patient shouldn't be eating," I said to the ward sister, who replied, "Her colostomy worked, and she was able to sit herself up and ask for breakfast. She looked so well, I gave her some."

One of the house officers with me asked why she was in the psychiatric hospital. I suggested she ask the patient how old she was. The patient stopped, thought for a moment, and then said, "A million years!" She also had other, more serious delusions but, as far as the operation was concerned, she made the quickest recovery from such an operation that I have ever seen. Two days later she was discharged back to the asylum and returned three months later for an uneventful closure of the colostomy by reversing the Hartmann's procedure.

One Saturday afternoon in the racing season, I was called to casualty to see a jockey who had fallen off his horse at the Warwick races and had been brought in with breathing difficulties. He was a famous jockey, and I knew who he was as soon as I saw him. He was severely distressed. Physical examination of his chest showed marked signs of crepitus under the skin, caused by air escaping from a tear in the lung that had spread to the subcutaneous tissues through the disruption of his chest wall. The injured side of the chest was much more expanded than the other, due to the air entering the pleural cavity through a rent in the lung, increasing in volume with each inspiration. Rapidly the pressure built up within the pleural cavity and pushed the trachea towards the opposite side of the chest. He had developed a classic tension pneumothorax.

This condition is associated with a fractured rib and gives the sensation of softness and bubbles under the skin. If a pneumothorax such as this is not treated immediately, a cardiac arrest rapidly follows, as the heart is also forced to shift by the increasing pressure of the tension of the air in the pleural cavity, so causing the great veins in the thorax to kink, reducing or stopping the venous blood flow into the heart.

When a large needle was inserted between the ribs, there was a satisfactory hiss of air escaping, relieving the pressure and enabling the patient to breathe freely again and a drain was then inserted. After X-rays confirming two fractured ribs, he was taken to a ward.

When I saw him next day he was comfortable, but not at all pleased about anything—the ward, the treatment, or me—a salutary lesson that a doctor must do what is necessary and not expect thanks. However, I decided not to place any bets on the horses he rode!

Mr Marsh was always extremely punctual and started all his lists exactly at the scheduled time. The time of starting was nine o'clock with "knife to skin." This meant that the anaesthetist had to have the patient asleep and on the operating table at the scheduled time. The surgical team had already been on the wards for an hour doing a ward round before arriving at the operating theatres in time to change and scrub, ready for the start of the list at nine o'clock exactly.

There was one occasion when it snowed and the young Australian anaesthetist scheduled to give the anaesthetics for Mr Marsh's list was late. He turned up at half past nine, much to Mr Marsh's annoyance. "Where have you been, Dr Ganter?" he asked. "I have been taking photographs of the snow," was the reply in a deep Australian accent. Mr Marsh laughed. He said to me afterwards that there was no point in his being cross with such a genuine excuse. Dr Ganter had never seen snow before.

Many was the time that I started operating at 9.00 a.m. and was still operating at midnight and sometimes on through the night on acute surgical emergencies that had come in during that day and night. Operating through the night was usually very peaceful, as there were few interruptions. The hospital was so quiet, and coming home at dawn on a summer's morning was refreshing. I have been asked if these long hours led to mistakes being made. I cannot remember a single time when I was even drowsy while working, either on the ward, in casualty, or in theatre. It was interesting and totally absorbing work, and I was constantly aware of my responsibility.

After two years of non-stop work for Mr Marsh I transferred to be the orthopaedic registrar at Warwick working for Messrs Duke and Tansy. This move was necessary to complete the job requirements needed before becoming eligible to sit the examination for fellowship of the Royal College of Surgeons of England (FRCS). This was an enjoyable job but not nearly as busy as the general surgical job I had been doing. The hours were nominally as long, but I was not called out nearly as frequently. I did miss the general surgery but learned a great deal of orthopaedics that proved very helpful a decade later. Amongst the orthopaedic operations I learned to do were lumbar discectomies and a prototype total hip replacement using the Ring prosthesis, which has long since been superseded. This latter operation was only successful for a short time, as the prosthetic ball and socket were both made of metal and tended to fuse, rendering the artificial hip immobile. It was soon replaced by Charnley's[2] hip prosthesis.

Problems come round again, for in 2012, another metal-on-metal prosthetic hip joint was manufactured and subsequently banned for the same reason as the Ring prosthesis. Sir John Charnley had a pub named after him in Standish near Wrightington Hospital, where he had carried out his pioneering work. It was simply called the "Sir John Charnley," probably the only pub named after a surgeon except for Lord Lister.

It was commonly said in surgical circles that somebody who had carried out a huge amount of surgery in a short time was said to be "overexperienced and undertrained." Having been awarded my fellowship of the Royal College of Surgeons in 1972, I began to look for a post at a London teaching hospital to rectify this sad state of affairs! There was nothing available at St Thomas's Hospital. However, a job for a post-fellowship registrar was advertised at the Middlesex Hospital and Medical School in the *British Journal of Medicine,* and so I applied. It was time to move on, although working for John Marsh at Warwick had been the best of times.

---

[2] Charnley John, The long-term results of low friction arthroplasty of the hip performed as a primary intervention. J Bone Joint Surg. Feb 1972 vol. 54-B no.1 61-76.

Table 1

Operating at Warwick Hospital, 1971-1973.

The author. aged 28-29, made detailed anatomical and surgical notes on operations, assisted at, then personally carried out, first under direct and then later indirect supervision. The date when some of the operations were first performed with assistance is noted.

Endocrine
Thyroidectomy, subtotal, 07/05/1971
Parotidectomy, superficial, 24/06/1971
Upper gastro-intestinal.
Gastrectomy, Billroth I for haematemesis, 05/06/1971
Vagotomy and pyloroplasty,
       HeinekeMickulicz, 13/06/1971
Trans-thoracic vagotomy, 23/06/1971
Gastro-enterostomy, 20/01/1971
Total gastrectomy,
       with oesophago-jejunal anastomosis. 09/03/1972
Heller's Operation,
       for atresia of the cardia, 26/10/1971
Vagotomy and antrectomy, 19/02/1972
Colorectal.
Right hemicolectomy,
       carcinoma of the caecum, 14/06/1971
Abdomino-perineal excision of the rectum, 12/07/1971
Haemorrhoidectomy.
Anal fistula operations.
Hepatobiliary Surgery.
Cholecystectomy.
Choledocho-duodenostomy, 01/12/1971
Cholecystectomy and exploration of the Common Bile Duct.
Vascular Surgery.
Amputation of toes, 10/06/1971
Syme's amputation, 01/12/1971
Lumbar sympathectomy, 06/10/1971
Peripheral embolectomy.
Above-knee and below-knee Amputations.

Urological Surgery
Pyelolithotomy, 19/07/1971
Millin's prostatectomy, 12/08/1971
Urethral bouginage.
Trans-vesical prostatectomy, 12/08/1971
Vasectomy.
Circumcision.
Paediatric surgery.
Closure of meningo-myelocoele, 21/06/1971
Insertion of Spitz-Holter valve, 13/09/1971
Hernia repairs.
Femoral hernia, 14/06/1971
Henry's Operation for bilateral inguinal hernias.
Bassini's inguinal hernia repair.
Incisional hernia repair.
Herniotomies.
Emergency General Surgery.
Exploratory laparotomies for haemorrhage, perforation,
      bowel obstruction etc.
Splenectomies.
Strangulated inguinal hernias.
Strangulated femoral hernias.
Tracheostomies.
Small bowel obstructions.
Colostomies.
Appendicectomies.
Closure of perforated peptic ulcers.
Emergency neuro-surgery.
Burr holes.
Raising cranial flaps.
Raising depressed cranial fractures.
Operations assisted at but not performed.
Saphenofemoral bypass graft.
Axillofemoral bypass graft.
Cervical sympathectomy.
Urinary diversion with an ileal conduit.
Total cystectomy.
Reconstruction of ano-rectal atresia.

CHAPTER 6

Surgical Registrar, the Middlesex Hospital, 1973–1975

An advertisement in the *British Medical Journal* called for applicants for the appointment of a post-fellowship surgical registrar at the Middlesex Hospital, which was cheek by jowl with Soho in London. The post was to work for Messrs Cecil Murray and William Slack, who were the consultants of a general surgical firm with a particular interest in endocrine and colorectal surgery respectively. Ten years later Mr Slack was knighted and appointed Serjeant Surgeon to HM the Queen (1983-1990).

The interview process was the norm at that time. There were no set questions, and any line of interest was followed by the interviewers. All the candidates stayed after being interviewed because the appointment of the successful candidate was always decided immediately after all interviews were completed. It was policy to invite the preferred candidate to come back into the interview room to confirm that he would accept the appointment. This, I learned later, when experienced at interviewing myself, was because candidates naturally applied for several jobs. If the successful candidate had, for example, an interview at another hospital the following day, he was expected to cancel that and any other subsequent interviews. The appointment had to be accepted the same day. All unsuccessful candidates were then counselled by a member of the selection committee about their interview and given encouragement and pointers for the future.

If in the event that the post was refused by the preferred candidate, then the next preferred candidate was still present and could be appointed. I remember one occasion when an appointment was made, and two days later the appointee rang to turn the job down, having received what he considered a better offer elsewhere. The consultants whose job he turned down were furious and complained to the General Medical Council (GMC). This was understandable, as any other suitable candidate had now gone, and the whole lengthy appointment process would have to be restarted. Meanwhile, the firm might well have gone weeks or months with the post unfilled. I was fortunate to be the candidate appointed.

So in March 1973, I was installed as the registrar on a general surgical firm in a London teaching hospital. This was indeed a moment of pride. The emergency registrar's on-call duties meant living away from home every fourth week from 9.00 a.m. on Monday morning until the next Monday evening. If on the Monday following the week's take there was a patient who had been admitted with an unresolved acute abdomen, for example, it was expected that the admitting registrar would continue to stay in residence at the hospital until the problem was resolved, either by the patient getting better or having an operation. This was in the interests of continuity of care, a principle with which I am in total agreement but that Professor Le Quesne took to its logical extreme conclusion. It would have been quite possible to hand over such a patient to the new surgical registrar on duty on the Monday morning then review the patient again together in the evening before departing for home, but this was not allowed.

At Warwick I had been on duty virtually all the time, but as home was only one hundred and fifty metres from the hospital, I could rest there whenever there was any lull in the work. The

Middlesex Hospital, being in the centre of London, was busy by day, but as all the commuters left for home at the end of the day, it was then very quiet, with few emergencies for the duty surgeons to look after or operate on during the night. It is a truism that when there is little to do, it takes more effort to do what has to be done. So a new emergency needed more effort to deal with it. The opposite is the case when the workload is heavy, for then another emergency arriving in casualty is just fitted into the emergency schedule and looked after. Under these circumstances, the extra effort needed to look after more patients causes no problems.

Thus the pace of life was very different from that in Warwick, enabling me to redress the balance of work experience against scholarship. This was not to foster a satisfactory work/life balance, a concept that in the early seventies had yet to be invented, but to avoid the sobriquet of being overexperienced and undertrained. It soon became apparent that where I had carried out hundreds of operations at Warwick, my new colleagues, who had stayed in the teaching hospital, had done many fewer in the same time. A new registrar attached to a surgical firm is assessed by his consultants, and it usually takes several months to get to know their trainee, gauge his ability, and develop confidence to allow him to operate on their patients both competently and safely. Fortunately, Mr Jeremy Wilson, the firm's senior registrar, had overall charge under the consultants and observing that I had experience, soon put me to work both operating and teaching. There were always five or six students to be taught clinical surgery, as well as younger doctors.

My time was well spent at the Middlesex. My reading of surgery deepened, and there was time to consider diseases and operations at length with regular clinical seminars and attendance at medical conferences, including the Association of Surgeons and the Surgical Research Society. It was an enjoyable time, with more contemplation to redress the balance in my training. The technical surgery that I had the opportunity to advance was in endocrine and colorectal surgery in particular. During the next two years, I learnt to operate on the thyroid, parathyroid, and adrenal glands. Mr Murray was a national expert in endocrine surgery and would operate weekly on patients with overactive parathyroid gland(s) who were referred from all over the south of England. The students were under the impression that an overactive parathyroid was more common than acute appendicitis! Parathyroidectomy was carried out in close collaboration with Dr O'Riodan, a distinguished endocrinologist and a pioneer in early diagnosis of hyperparathyroidism. He carried out a battery of tests on these patients preoperatively, not only to confirm the diagnosis, but also to attempt to locate which of the four parathyroid glands was responsible for the over-secretion of parathormone. This latter endeavour was still in its infancy, but it was a goal that might greatly assist the surgeon in finding the often secretive abnormal gland(s) at operation. However it was not successful. So all these techniques were gradually abandoned, as it became apparent at that time, that the best way to find a parathyroid adenoma was to find a surgeon who could find a parathyroid adenoma!

Localising a parathyroid adenoma can be difficult at operation, as noted above. The lower pair of glands are usually found in intimate contact with the lobes of the thyroid and adjacent to the recurrent laryngeal nerves, which innervate the vocal cords. Any damage of these delicate nerves, which have the width of about a thread, can paralyse the larynx, causing serious problems with speech and singing. I studied Mr Murray's meticulous technique of operating in detail when assisting him. Only once in my later career did I inadvertently bruise a recurrent laryngeal nerve, which fortunately did not disable the patient, but it caused me much anxiety until full recovery had taken place.

Another opportunity was to increase my skills in colorectal surgery under the supervision of Mr Slack. Every week the rectal clinic was held in the oldest outpatients department in the hospital. It comprised a long hall with curtained examination cubicles down the whole of one side. Patients were ushered into the cubicles by the clinic nurses through doors that gave access from an outside corridor into each cubicle. The nurse then told the patients which garments to take off. This clinic was always very quiet; all the doctors, nurses, and patients talked in whispers.

Having taken a history and carried out a detailed examination, including internal examination and rigid sigmoidoscopy, each member of the surgical team returned to his own desk. There to write up the notes and arrange, after discussion with Mr Slack, investigations or list the patient for operation. The desks were in a row facing the examination cubicles and were contemporary with Charles Dickens's time, being desks with a sloping top that the user had to stand at in order to write. They must have been used by clerks a century before.

One of the most important successes of the clinic was from the routine rectal examination and sigmoidoscopy. This was so well organised that it did not, on average, add more than a couple of minutes to the overall examination and meant that all rectal carcinomas were diagnosed at the first consultation. The biopsy taken for histology at the same time usually confirmed the diagnosis. The time between first being seen in the clinic and definitive operation was at most three weeks. Also, a large number of cases of inflammatory bowel disease were diagnosed, enabling medical treatment to be started immediately.

Any patient needing further examination of the bowel had a barium enema booked and was reviewed, with the result in due course. Apart from the absence of the scribe's desks, I copied the organisation of running this rectal clinic when I was a consultant.

Some patients had venereal disease and were transferred to the special clinic the same day. As noted earlier, the Middlesex Hospital was close to Soho, so there was a constant traffic of patients to and from the rectal clinic to the special clinic and vice versa. The special clinic is now called the genito-urinary clinic, a name for a more utilitarian age.

In Mr Slack's operating theatres, there was much new and interesting happening. It was the era of Sir Alan Parks and the development of the continent ileostomy. Patients who had been cured of ulcerative colitis by a total excision of the colon and rectum must have an ileostomy to evacuate their bowel. However, Mr Slack was beginning to offer his patients a continent ileostomy. In the standard ileostomy, the end of the terminal ileum is brought out onto the abdominal wall and formed into a spout, so the liquid bowel contents can drain directly into a bag. With the continent ileostomy, a pouch is fashioned from the terminal loop of ileum, with the final portion of the ileum inverted to form a valve that prevents any leakage of bowel contents. The patient then has control of emptying the pouch by inserting a catheter into it and draining the contents at a suitable place and time. I was taught how to form a pouch or reservoir from small bowel. The theory was good, but the continent ileostomy itself was never really a very successful operation at that time. Learning the craft of making pouches from small bowel using several different techniques was of great use a few years later. It was the repetition and confidence gained in carrying out a procedure under supervision that was so valuable. All the pouches were sewn by hand.

Another novel advance was in the treatment of cancer of the rectum with fewer total excisions of the rectum, thus sparing many patients the otherwise inevitable permanent colostomy. It is now technically possible to excise tumours that are growing very close to the anal margin and anastomose the sigmoid colon just above the anus, thus maintaining bowel continuity and avoiding a colostomy. When I was a student and a houseman, I was taught that the only way to give a patient the best chance of a cure from cancer of the rectum was by carrying out a wide block dissection of all the associated lymphatics, including the lymph nodes up to the origin of the inferior mesenteric artery. To accomplish this, it was thought that there must be fifteen centimetres of normal rectum from the anal margin to the lower edge of the cancer. Five of those 15 cm were excised with the growth to ensure that the cancer was completely removed, leaving a cuff of normal rectum. This remaining 10 cm of the rectum maintained a functioning reservoir, so the patient retained normal sensation of rectal fullness and full control over bowel evacuation. Cancers closer than 15 cm to the anal margin were excised by removing the whole rectum in an abdomino-perineal excision of the rectum (AP) as described in the previous chapter. The possibility of safely excising a rectal cancer much closer to the anus was beginning to be realised from information learned by excising benign villous papillomas of the rectum, which sometimes involved the rectal mucosa down to the anus.

Operations for the removal of a benign villous papilloma of the rectum abutting the anal margin involved stripping the mucosa carrying the papilloma from the rectum, leaving a large area of the underlying smooth muscle exposed. This gradually healed with mucosa growing in from the surrounding edges. This proceedure did not disrupt the normal rectal sensation for flatus and faeces, thus a normally functioning rectum was maintained. This was a novel finding, as it had been assumed previously that proprioceptors in the mucosa itself were essential for normal sensation to maintain continence. Gradually surgeons were moving closer and closer to the anal margin on excising a cancer. Thus the sigmoid colon could now be brought down and sutured to the anus, while satisfactory control was maintained in most patients. However, it was technically difficult to perform this low anastomosis in some men, due to a very narrow pelvis, which made it impossible to get a good enough view to hand sew the colon to the anus. In these patients the much more radical operation of abdomino-perineal excision of the rectum remained the operation of choice. There were no stapling devices, radiotherapy, or chemotherapy for cancer of the rectum at that time.

The first case of potential litigation I came across was on a routine ward round when reviewing a young American woman in her twenties. She had the misfortune to have been caught between a car and a wall and while still standing had been forcibly rolled between the two. This had resulted in a very serious injury that I had repaired ten days before. Now she was ready for discharge from hospital. When I told her that she could go for convalescence, the young woman said that her lawyer had been to see her and advised her to stay in hospital for another week. It transpired that the extra stay would increase the compensation paid to her, and it was apparent that my patient thought that this would be such a large sum that she would never need to work again. I politely explained that her treatment was not directed by her legal adviser and discharged her as planned.

The injury this woman had sustained had resulted in a fractured pelvis. Worse, it had split and disrupted her anal sphincter. I used the technique of anal repair pioneered by Mr Aubrey York Mason[1]—having had the privilege to watch him operate at St Thomas's Hospital in 1969 and recently having carried out the same operation under Mr Slack's supervision—and I was able to successfully repair this woman's anal sphincter.

Mr Yorke Mason had devised this operation to give direct surgical access for repair of iatrogenic vesico-rectal fistulas sometimes caused by Millin's open prostatectomy. It needed meticulous attention to restoring the anatomical sphincter layer by layer. As an aside, it is interesting to note that the anus was, I believe, the last organ in the body that yielded to surgical repair. It was accomplished by Yorke Mason only after the first heart transplant was carried out by Professor Christiaan Barnard in December 1967.

---

[1] Mason, York A. Surgical access to the rectum, a trans-sphincteric exposure. Proc. Roy. Soc. Med. 1970, 63:91-94.

Vascular surgery at the Middlesex was pioneered by Mr Adrian Marsden, a brilliant surgeon who was also a noted linguist. When he was to operate on an aortic aneurysm, there would be only one case for an all-day operating list. The operation was listed as "abdominal aortic aneurysm resection." Once exposed, the aneurysm was carefully dissected out as far as possible. It was not always possible to complete this excision. After about three hours operating, the team stopped for a break and had lunch. After lunch they returned and finished the dissection and finally sewed in a synthetic graft to bridge the gap in the aorta and restore blood flow into the lower abdomen and legs. This was a very taxing and time-consuming operation for both the patient and the surgical team.

The style in which lunches were served to the surgeons in the operating theatres at the Middlesex Hospital came straight out of the inter-war years. Attached to the operating theatre was a separate dining room and kitchen. Two long tables were covered with fresh white tablecloths, and place settings were formally laid. Huge jugs of water and orange juice were placed on the tables, and although there was no menu, three courses were served by a waitress. These meals were a treat and a wonderful opportunity to discuss the operations being done that day with detailed talk of techniques and interesting and difficult procedures. It was indeed a pleasure and an inspiration. Needless to say, this dining room was closed a few years later—a great loss of a semi-formal setting where surgeons could sit down to talk in depth about their work and exchange ideas.

Time was rolling on, and the end of my appointment at the Middlesex was now in sight, and I was wondering how to pursue my career. There was no set pathway to becoming a consultant surgeon in the seventies. I liked the idea of spending some time in research with a view to obtaining a doctorate in medicine, a plan suggested to me by Professor Michael Hobsley. Professor Hobsley held a personal chair in surgery at the Middlesex Hospital in the academic department of surgery and had a laboratory in the hospital, from which a steady flow of papers were published in the best medical journals. To join Professor Hobsley's research team it was necessary to have external funding.

I applied to the Wellcome Trust for a two-year fellowship with a description of the proposed research, which in my case involved study of gastric secretion in relation to ulcers of the duodenum and the effectiveness of operations to cure this disease in individual patients. My application was followed by a long and detailed interview at the Wellcome Trust, after which I was awarded a grant for two years at the same salary that I had been receiving as a surgical registrar. It was a great privilege to have been selected to become a Wellcome research fellow, and I was delighted. The only drawback was how much I would miss the clinical work, especially the operating.

So with pay secured, when my contract as surgical registrar expired I moved into a small office in the basement of the hospital to carry out research. It was very exciting, and I was lucky that Professor Hobsley would be my supervisor while I worked towards producing a thesis worthy of presenting to Oxford University for a doctorate of medicine.

CHAPTER 7

Wellcome Research Fellow at the Middlesex Hospital, 1975-1977.

The first day that I was installed in my new office, I was rung from Professor Le Quesne's outpatient clinic to ask me to take the place of one of his staff, who had been unable to come to assist that day. My natural instinct was to oblige, but I had noticed while I was working as a surgical registrar that a colleague who was supposed to be doing research seemed to spend all his time filling in for others, to no particular benefit to himself. My contract with the Wellcome Trust was quite specific on this point and allowed only four hours a week for either clinical work or teaching. I had decided I could best use this time to teach students. There followed a conversation on the phone, in which I explained why I could not join the clinic. I was a bit worried after that, but to my relief I was never asked again, so my contract was respected by the professor, for which I was grateful.

The reason for the wide academic interest in peptic ulcers in the mid-twentieth century was not only medical and scientific but also economic. It is extraordinary to look back to 1973, for example, when the disease was so common that 1.8 million working days were lost due to the ill health ulcers caused in Britain (Dr K. D. Barden).[1]

Statistics from all sources indicate that 10% or more of the Western populations were afflicted by the disease at some time of their lives and it accounted for approximately 10% of all adult admissions to general hospitals (Professor M. J. S. Langman).[2] Peptic ulcer is the generic term for benign ulcers of the stomach (gastric ulcers) and duodenum (duodenal ulcers); where an ulcer is referred to in this chapter, it is always a duodenal ulcer.

The main symptoms of the disease were indigestion and upper abdominal pain, which was often severe. Since it was a chronic condition, it frequently lasted for years with long relapses and remissions. As the years passed, the remissions often got shorter and less frequent. Complications were common.

These complications include perforation of the ulcer, which occurs as the disease extends beyond the lining of the duodenum and penetrates the muscular wall of the organ. Thus weakened, the base of the ulcer gives way, and the acidic contents of the stomach leak into the peritoneum, causing acute peritonitis with excruciating pain. Without treatment peritonitis is usually fatal. Another complication is haemorrhage. The bleeding is caused by erosion of an artery that has been exposed in the base of the ulcer, which can be severe and life-threatening. Long-term ulceration of the duodenum can also lead to extensive scar tissue forming around it. The resulting narrowing or stenosis can cause copious and daily vomiting.

In 1910, the brilliant Russian physiologist Ivan Pavlov[5] proved that stimulation of the vagus nerves (vagi) in dogs caused secretion of acid by the stomach. The left and right vagus nerves arise in the brain and are numbered as the tenth cranial nerves. These nerves gather into two trunks on the lower oesophagus, one in front and one behind, and on passing into the abdominal cavity they divide into branches to innervate the stomach and other organs.

TABLE.2

	Gastric ulcer Perforated only	Gastric ulcer Total	Duodenal ulcer Perforated only	Duodenal ulcer Total
1959- 1962	2,567	26,669	5,430	38,520
1963-1966	1,887	21,399	5,271	37,948
1967-1970	1,700	19,560	5,259	37,002
1971-1974	1,478	16,895	4,853	33,696
Percentage change from 1959-1962 to 1971-1974	-42.3%	-36.6%	-10.6%	-12.5%

Table 2. *The table above reproduced from Professor M. J. S. Langman's[3] book shows the estimated number of in-patients aged fifteen or more who were admitted to hospital on account of peptic ulceration and also the number of these who had perforated their peptic ulcer between 1959 and 1974. Data is from hospital in-patient enquiries in England and Wales. (Revised and updated).[4] These data give an idea of the scale of the problem caused by peptic ulcer disease and the relevance of research into its cause and treatment.*

In 1922, Laterjet[6] recorded that when the human vagi were divided, there was a reduction in the subsequent hydrochloric acid secretion by the stomach. An excess of gastric acid had for many years been assumed to be responsible for the continuation, if not the cause, of ulcers.[7] Supporting evidence was the increase in the acid-secreting parietal cells of the stomach from the normal level of about a billion cells to two billion by the time a patient had suffered from a chronic duodenal ulcer for nine years. These considerations led, in 1943, to the reintroduction in the United States by Dragstedt and Owens[8] of a transthoracic vagotomy to divide these nerves at the level of the lower oesophagus as a treatment for duodenal ulcer by reducing the acid secreted into the stomach and so allow the ulcer to heal.

The most powerful evidence in support of the efficacy of vagotomy in treating duodenal ulcers came from the very high cure rate achieved by many surgeons. The earliest and commonest operation was the truncal vagotomy (TV) as described above, which not only denervated the parasympathetic nerve supply to the stomach but also the liver, small bowel, and ascending colon. In a meta-analysis[9] of 4,470 patients undergoing TV, 93% were permanently cured. This left a proven and suspected recurrence rate of 7%. There was, however, concern about the wide variation of recurrent ulcers between different surgeons, ranging from 1% to 20%. Virtually all the patients undergoing TV in the forties and early fifties had scarring and narrowing of the duodenum due to years of suffering from their ulcers. With a scarred duodenum, it was essential to enable the stomach to empty properly, and one of a number of drainage operations was carried out at the same time as the vagotomy. By the seventies, the most common operation used to achieve this was a pyloroplasty, in which the opening of the stomach into the duodenum was enlarged. The combined operation of vagotomy and pyloroplasty was usually referred to as a V&P. By the late seventies, surgeons were operating on patients at an earlier stage of the disease, often before scarring had occurred. If the absence of duodenal scarring was confirmed at operation, the duodenum no longer needed to be enlarged, and so a pyloroplasty was unnecessary.

Operations were then devised to avoid a truncal vagotomy (TV), which cuts the parasympathetic nerve supply not only to the target area of the parietal or acid-secreting cells of the stomach but also other organs, as noted above. A selective vagotomy (SV) was devised to preserve those branches of the vagi that innervate the liver and the gut, while still denervating the whole stomach. Finally a proximal gastric vagotomy (PGV), also called a highly selective vagotomy,[10] was devised. In this operation, only the nerve fibres supplying the acid-secreting parietal cells of the stomach were divided. This aimed to also preserve the nerves supplying the antrum of the stomach. The antrum has no acid-secreting cells but propels the stomach contents on into the duodenum. By preserving its nerve supply, the normal contractions of the antrum will continue, and so maintain satisfactory emptying of the stomach. The rate of recurrent ulcers following these last two operations was no different in the early analysis from that quoted above for V&P, but it was found several years later to be higher.

It seemed inescapable that the commonest cause of recurrent duodenal ulcer was an incomplete or inadequate vagotomy, where some fibres of the vagi supplying the acid-secreting parietal cells of the stomach remain intact after surgery. Even a few tiny nerve fibres undivided resulted in sufficient acid secretion to continue after the operation, thus leading to a recurrence of the ulcer. As early as 1948, Hollander[11] devised a postvagotomy gastric secretion test to see if the operation was adequate. The stimulus to assess residual acid secretion in postvagotomy patients was a calibrated injection of insulin. This became known as the "Hollander test," and in spite of Hollander's own assertion that "the test cannot be used to prognosticate clinical results of vagotomy,"[12] it was still the standard test[13,14] to assess the adequacy of vagotomy in the midseventies.

A significant reason for the unreliability of the Hollander test was technical. It took no account of the normal flow of gastric juice from the stomach into the duodenum during a lengthy test in which gastric juice was sucked out of the stomach. These "losses" of gastric juice from the analysis were ignored, despite the fact that the errors so caused could be substantial,[15] being as much as 20%. Reflux of alkaline juice from the duodenum was also not corrected for. Another cause of unreliability was that the Hollander test used the patient's own resting or basal secretion as a control to make the comparison with the subsequent insulin-stimulated secretion. Basal or resting secretion of the stomach is known to vary in everybody when measured several times on different occasions,[16] making it unreliable as a standard against which to measure change.

The insulin-stimulated gastric-secretion test used at the Middlesex Hospital had been pioneered by Professor Hobsley and his associates. They developed reproducible methods of measuring pyloric losses[17,18] and reflux of alkaline juice from the duodenum.[19,20,21] The actual volume of gastric juice collected was then corrected for these factors. This test, which I suggest should be called the "Hobsley test," was the most accurate gastric-secretion test of that time and possibly the most reproducible ever devised in humans. Having established the validity and reproducibility of the collection of gastric juice, Professor Hobsley focused on the accurate measurement of insulin and histamine-stimulated secretion of gastric acid and its relationship to duodenal ulcer disease in patients.

Before carrying out tests on patients, it was necessary to secure the permission of the hospital ethics committee, whose rules were strict concerning patient safety and the potential value of the investigation. Signed informed consent from the patient was always obtained well in advance. The actual tests on the patients lasted about three and a half hours and involved injecting a carefully measured dose of insulin. Insulin injected into the bloodstream naturally lowers the blood sugar level in the test subject and induces a feeling of hunger. This triggers a reflex from the brain causing the vagi to stimulate the parietal cells to secrete acid into stomach in preparation for digesting food. It had been proved in earlier experiments that a measured dose of insulin achieves the same secretion of acid in a controlled and repeatable manner in any individual patient. By comparison, histamine infusion directly stimulates the parietal cells to secrete the maximum volume of acid possible, as no neural reflex is involved and the test is likewise repeatable in a single individual.

Using Hobsley's test, gastric juice was collected (after insulin stimulation) in sequential aliquots every ten minutes by continual suction on a tube passed into the patient's stomach. Each sample was bottled and labelled. After the test, all the samples were analysed in the laboratory by Mr Pete Whitfield, who calculated for each sample the losses of gastric juice from the stomach and reflux into the stomach from the duodenum. After making these corrections, the final figure of gastric juice (V_G) in each sample was available for calculations.

When I joined Professor Hobsley's laboratory, this work had already been completed for a paper, published by my colleague Richard Faber[22] in 1975, titled, "A New Interpretation of the Insulin Test." This paper established new criteria, based on the comparison of insulin-stimulated gastric juice in individuals after vagotomy to the range of insulin-stimulated secretion in a large group of patients with duodenal ulcers who had not had an operation. These data were collected only from men. At that time, the data from women were not comparable with that of men. However, at last there was a predictive test to check postoperatively the completeness of the vagotomy to the acid-secreting cells of the stomach in men. This information was not of help to the individual patient who had undergone this operation, but it did test the skills of the surgeon, who could then adjust the operating technique to improve the results of future operations.

The first objective of my thesis was to develop Faber's new interpretation of the insulin test, so it could be applied equally to all individuals of whatever stature and whether male or female. As already noted, the increased predictive value of recurrence is of small comfort to the individual patient who has undergone vagotomy.

The second aim of the thesis was to investigate the accuracy of a peroperative test to check for adequacy of vagotomy by using the electrical stimulation test of Burge and Vane (1958).[23] If it could be reliably demonstrated during an operation that the vagotomy was inadequate, then the surgeon would have the opportunity to remedy the deficiency immediately, to the great advantage of the patient. I carried out the Burge test in the latter part of my time as a research fellow, as much work had been needed to correlate the secretion of men and women.

The technique of the Burge test may be of interest. A wide-bore, fairly stiff plastic tube was passed by the anaesthetist down the oesophagus into the stomach. A circular clamp with electrodes, which was designed to open, was then clamped round the intra-abdominal portion of the oesophagus and carefully closed to secure an airtight seal between the clamp and the plastic tube, with the lower oesophagus between. A soft clamp was then applied across the antrum of the stomach to stop any air or fluid entering the duodenum (figure 1). Air was then gently pumped into the stomach through the plastic tube to distend the stomach, and the upper end of the tube was sealed by a pressure-recording device. A low current was passed through the electrodes in the clamp to stimulate any residual vagus nerve fibres, which all carry not only secretor fibres but also motor fibres. If any fibres were still present, electrical stimulation would cause contraction of the connected stomach's muscular tissue, resulting in an increase in the intragastric pressure. Any rise in pressure indicated that the operation was incomplete (figure 2). In these circumstances, after removal of the apparatus, the surgeon would carry out a further search for the errant fibres.

As there is no gender difference between the sexes where the stomach is concerned, the size of the individual should correlate to the size of their stomach within. In turn, the volume of acid secreted should also correlate with the size of the stomach. If all subjects of these tests, both male and female, could be standardised for size, a direct comparison of the acid each secreted could also be standardised by the same factor, making accurate correlation possible.

Earlier work in 1952 by Cox[24] and in 1964 by Baron[25] found "no consistent relationship between stomach size, age, or body size," although by 1969, Baron[26] was able to show correlations for histamine-stimulated acid output with body weight and lean body mass in male patients with duodenal ulcers. In 1971, Hassan and Hobsley[27] found much higher correlations between stature and gastric secretion in response to histamine infusion, using several indices of stature, including lean body mass (LBM), height, weight, and body surface area. The best correlations were found with LBM and height; but only applied to data from men. As no useful correlation could be found combining the data from both men and women,[28,29] the studies on women were excluded.[30]

FIGURE 1

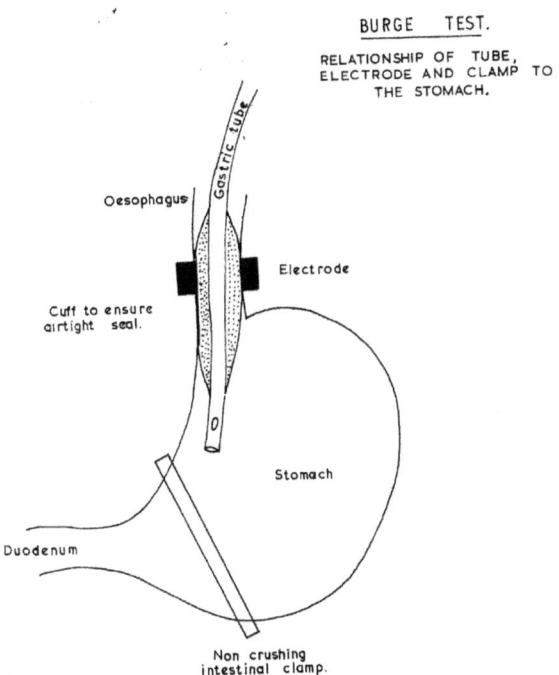

Figure 1. *Schematic diagram showing the Burge test apparatus in the stomach. Results of tracings are shown in figure 2*

FIGURE 2

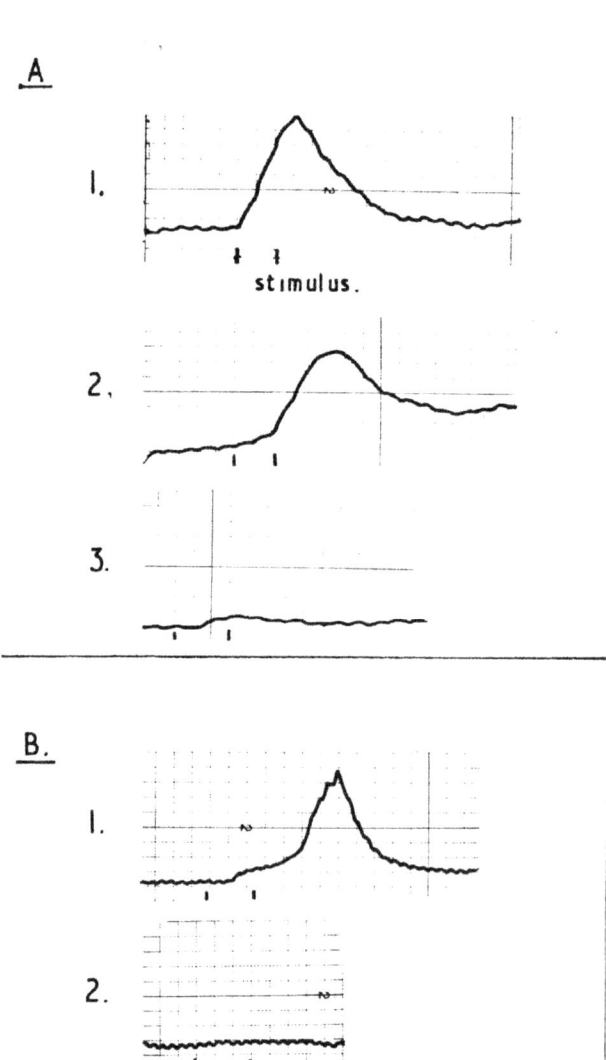

Figure 2. *Burge test tracings taken during the operation.*

Patient A.
1. *Prevagotomy response to electrical stimulation shows a high rise in pressure.*
2. *Following vagotomy stimulation still shows a significant rise in pressure indicating an inadequate vagotomy.*
3. *After a further search for nerve fibres this tracing was recorded. In the first five of these tests, this tiny rise in pressure was considered to show that the vagotomy was adequate. The subsequent postoperative Hobsley's insulin test showed that the vagotomy was inadequate in this group of patients. All subsequent operations involved the diligent search by the surgeon for all tiny vagal nerve fibres running down the terminal oesophagus, to ensure the vagotomy was complete.*

Patient B.
1. *Prevagotomy tracing following electrical stimulation.*
2. *Postvagotomy tracing shows no response to stimulation and is deemed adequate, which was confirmed at the postvagotomy Hobsley's insulin test.*

If it was possible, by using Hobsley's insulin test, to find a predictive correlation for developing a recurrent ulcer in combined data collected from both men and women following vagotomy, this would be a significant step forward.

I collected data on the weight and height of all patients undergoing Hobsley's insulin test. Because in the seventies there were a significant minority of overweight people, height proved to be a very much better measure of stature than weight. The apparent difference between men's and women's secretions was confirmed in uncorrected samples of gastric juice. However, it was only when these samples were corrected for gastric losses and duodenal reflux, and then adjusted to a standard height, that the statistical difference between the gastric secretion of men and women was eliminated.

The main findings of my research were, first, that gastric secretion data of both men and women could be correlated. This was achieved by using Hobsley's insulin test and correcting all the data of both sexes to a standard height. This validated the new interpretation[31] of the insulin test to accurately predict those individuals who would develop a recurrent ulcer following their vagotomy. Second, the use of the Burge test during the operation increased the success of the operation in each individual patient, and this therapeutically useful exercise was confirmed by using Hobsley's insulin test postoperatively, which showed if the vagotomy[32] was adequate.

During my two years as research fellow, I carried out nearly two hundred gastric-secretion tests to collect data for my thesis and add to the considerable database already built by Professor Hobsley and my predecessors. The seventies were only at the dawn of the electronic age, and statistical calculations took an age, as the only electronic help our laboratory had was a Wang calculator. The Wang was considered very sophisticated, but all the data had to be fed in by hand for every calculation. The calculations for my thesis took three months of long days to complete. Two years later, in 1978, one of the examiners for my thesis asked me to recheck some of the calculations. My heart sank, as I did not have the time to spare. However, by then I was working at the University of Leicester, and I was able to use their new mainframe computer. The exercise that had taken me three months to complete now took only a day and a half, and most of that time was spent entering the raw data. The calculations themselves took about an hour, and all the graphs that had originally been drawn laboriously by hand for my actual thesis were now beautifully printed automatically.

I have before me a copy of the fortieth edition of *Gray's Anatomy*, published in 2008, which notes that the anterior vagus lying on the oesophagus as it enters the abdomen from the thorax is formed mainly from fibres from the left vagus and is often in two or three strands. There is no indication that the posterior vagus is anything other than a single trunk before dividing into gastric and coeliac branches. The Middlesex work shows that the vagus varies enormously in its lower oesophageal section. Often, not just two trunks with only two or three branches are formed, but each vagus nerve can be subdivided into a sheaf of nerves.

These findings had significant consequences for patients undergoing vagotomy. Surgeons had for years excised a centimetre section of the main trunks of these nerves and considered the operation complete, whereas the tests outlined above show this not to be so in a minority of patients. In practice, therefore, to complete the operation successfully, the lower 2–5 cm of the oesophagus needs to be meticulously stripped of all nerve fibres.

I very much enjoyed my time as a research fellow at the Middlesex Hospital Medical School. It was good to lead an academic life for a couple of years, immersed in science and being one of Professor Hobsley's research team. Working as a scientist gave practical experience of the scientific method and evaluation of others' research. This was not, of course, the end of the endeavour to successfully treat patients afflicted by a major chronic illness in those days. Great changes were beginning to take place.

FIGURE 3

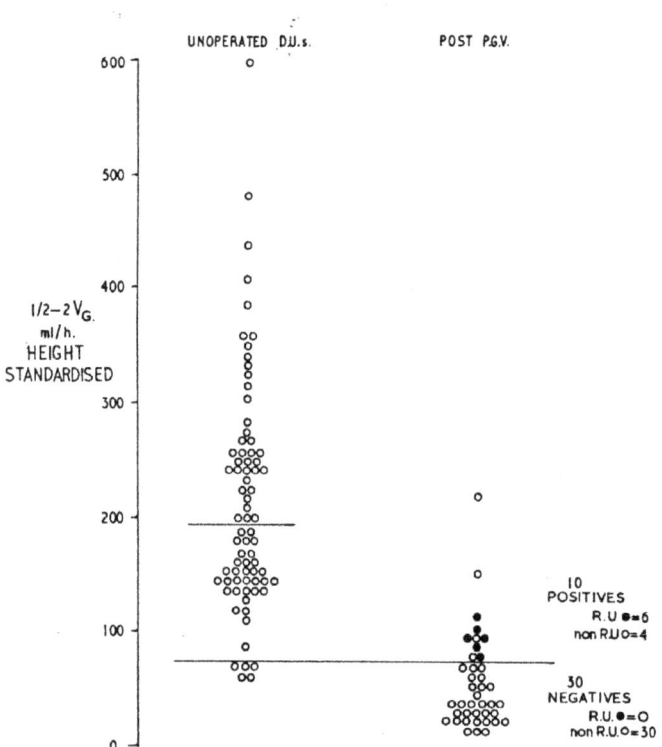

FIGURE 3. The figure above has been drawn to illustrate an analysis using Hobsley's insulin test in patients before and after undergoing proximal gastric vagotomy (PGV) without peroperative Burge testing. The left-hand column shows the preoperative volumes of insulin stimulated gastric secretion in millilitres (Hobsley's test) in 73 patients with chronic duodenal ulcers. The transverse line towards the bottom of the diagram indicates the lower 5 percentile level of secretion of these patients before operation. The right-hand column shows the result of Hobsley's insulin test carried out within six weeks of their vagotomy in forty patients. The right-hand column shows significant

reduction in the volume of acid secreted in all these post vagotomy patients. During close follow-up of 39 months, 10 patients' secretion was above the lower 5 percentile of secretion of the unoperated patients and of these, 6 developed a recurrent ulcer (black circles). None of the thirty below the preoperative lower 5 percentile developed a recurrent ulcer, open circles. The test was a first in accurately separating those patients who went on to develop a recurrence, but was disappointing in the fact that the rate of inadequate vagotomy was 15%. But it did confirm that the results of PGV were not as successful as TV. These results led to testing with the peroperative Burge test with improved results.

In 1976, the drug Cimetidine, an H_2 receptor antagonist, was marketed in the United Kingdom. James W. Black was awarded a deserved Nobel Prize in Medicine for his work in manufacturing what was probably the earliest designer drug in the literal sense. It was synthesised specifically to block the histamine$_2$ (H_2) receptors on the acid secreting parietal cells of the stomach. Cimetidine prevents histamine from activating acid secretion and so significantly reduces its output. This treatment could alleviate the symptoms caused by a duodenal ulcer, but when the drug was stopped, a relapse was the usual result. However, the necessity for surgery as a treatment of duodenal ulcer was now beginning to go into decline.

Helicobacter pylori were rediscovered in the stomach and duodenum in 1979 by J. Robin Warren, then in collaboration with Barry J. Marshall; they considered this bacterium to be the principle cause of peptic ulcer. This cause and effect was dramatically proved in 1984, when Barry Marshall swallowed the contents of a Petri dish of H. pylori and rapidly developed a severe gastritis, which was proved by endoscopy, biopsy, and culture to be caused by it. As supporting evidence from other researchers accumulated, antibiotic treatment of patients with peptic ulcer became the standard. The antibiotics are always prescribed with an acid-suppressing drug,

Omeprazole, a proton pump inhibitor first released in the United States in 1989. Drs Warren and Marshall also received a well-deserved Nobel Prize.

These seismic changes can be traced in the record of V&P operations I carried out as a consultant general surgeon in chapter 10/table 10. Between 1980 and 1985, the number of vagotomy and pyloroplasty operations averaged twelve a year. This was considerably fewer than in my registrar days in Warwick, when it seemed that there was a patient for this operation on every operating list. In 1990, the number of operations I carried out had fallen to five in that year, and in 1995, only one vagotomy was done, and none thereafter. Although Warren and Marshall frequently complained that their views were ignored, in fact, it only took ten years for elective surgery for duodenal ulcer disease to cease following their discovery.

Surgery is no longer the treatment of choice for duodenal ulcer. Now treatment by antibiotics and acid-suppressing drugs is the treatment of choice. This is a very satisfactory exchange for patients. This whole story represents an excellent example of the scientific method in action. The result is that patients are now cured by antibiotics administered by their general practitioners, rather than by a difficult operation. However, it must be remembered that before Warren and Marshall's discovery, the great majority of patients who underwent surgery for chronic duodenal ulcers were cured by the operation. The small percentage not cured by surgery or who developed serious long-term complications—caused by bile reflux or the "dumping syndrome"—had a difficult time and required further surgery, usually a partial gastrectomy. It must also be noted that the majority of patients with duodenal ulcer were not operated on. The trace of this can also be seen in my records in chapter 10/table 10 under "revision gastrectomy." This operation was no longer needed after 1990, as no further V&Ps were carried out. It must be noted that I inherited most of the patients in this group, who had had their vagotomy before my appointment as a consultant.

Thus, Warren and Marshall postulated a new theory for the cause of a duodenal ulcer disease. The medical and surgical establishments were interested but rightly sceptical. Many theories in the past that have been rushed into practice have been false dawns, to the detriment of patients and embarrassment of the profession. However, in this case the new treatment was validated by other workers and then became generally accepted. A scientific advance had taken place. However, a debate continues as to the cause of duodenal ulcers, because in some parts of the world duodenal ulcers occur without H. pylori infection.

My Wellcome fellowship was for a fixed term of two years, which meant that the money ran out on a fixed date. Six months before the end of the contract, I started the search for the next job. For career progression, the next appointment should be as a senior registrar, the last step before being eligible to apply for a post of consultant surgeon. Looking for a new job was interesting but not straightforward, as surgical training was carved out by the individual aspirant as opportunity presented itself. After searching around, I was fortunate to be appointed to a lectureship in surgery at the new medical school in Leicester. I was awarded my Doctorate of Medicine from Oxford University in 1980.

References

1. Bardan, K. D., Williamson, M., Royston, C., Lyon, C. Admission rates for peptic ulcer disease in Trent region, UK: a changing pattern a changing disease. Journal of Digestive and Liver Diseases. 2004: 577–588.
2. Langman, M. J. S. *The Epidemiology of chronic digestive diseases.* Chapter 2: Edward Arnold (Publishers) Ltd., London, 1979.

3. —. *The Epidemiology of Chronic Digestive Diseases*. Chapter 2. Edward Arnold (Publishers) Ltd., 1979.
4. Brown, R. C., M. J. S. Langman, and P. M. Lambert. "Hospital Admissions for Peptic Ulcer 1958-1972." *British Medical Journal* 1 (1976): 35–37.
5. Pavlov, I. P. *The Work of Digestive Glands*. Translated by W. H. Thompson.: (Publishers) Charles Griffin and Co., Ltd. London, 1910.
6. Laterjet, M. A. "Resections des Neufs de l'Estomac: Technique Operative Resultats Clinique." *Bull. Acad. Med.* 87 (1922): 681.
7. Kay, A. W. "Memorial Lecture: An Evaluation of Gastric Acid Excretion Tests." *Gastroenterology* 53 (1967): 834–841.
8. Dragstedt, C. R., and F. M. Owen, Jr. "Supradiaphragmatic Division of the Vagus Nerve Treatment of Duodenal Ulcer." *Proc. Soc. Exp. Med* 53 (1943): 152–154.
9. Goligher, J. C., and C. N. Pulvertaft. "Comparisons of Different Operations." In *After Vagotomy*, edited by J. A. Williams and A. G. Cox, chapter 8.(Publisher) Butterworth, London, 1969.
10. Johnston, D., and A. R. Wilkinson. "Highly Selective Vagotomy without a Drainage Procedure in the Treatment of Duodenal Ulcer." *British J Surg.* 54 (1970): 831–833.
11. Hollander, F. "The Insulin Test for the Presence of Intact Nerve Fibres after Vagal Operations for Peptic Ulcers." *Gastroenterology* 7 (1946): 607–614.
12. Weinstein, V. A., and F. Hollander. "Is the Insulin Test Always Reliable?" *Gastroenterology* 14 (1950): 586–590.
13. Kronborg, O., and P. Madsen. "A Controlled Randomised Trial of Highly Selective Vagotomy versus Selective Vagotomy and Pyloroplasty in the Treatment of Duodenal Ulcer." *Gut* 16 (1975): 268–271.

14. Kennedy, T., D. Johnston, et al. "Proximal Gastric Vagotomy: Interim Results of a Randomised Trial." *Brit. Med. J.* 2 (1975): 301–303.

15. Farmer, D. A., et al. "The Effects of Various Procedures upon the Acidity of the Gastric Contents of Ulcer Patients." *Annals of Surgery* 134 (1951): 319–331.

16. Baron, J. H., and J. Alexander-Williams. In *Recent Advances in Surgery*, page 172, Ed. Selwyn Taylor, (Publisher) Churchill Livingstone, Edinburgh and London, 1973.

17. Hobsley, M., and W. Silen. "Use of an Inert Marker (phenol red) to Improve Accuracy in Gastric Secretion Studies." *Gut* 10 (1969): 787–795.

18. Hobsley, M., and W. Silen. "The Relation between the Rate of Production of Gastric Juice and Its Electrolyte Concentration." *Clinical Science* 39 (1970): 61–75.

19. Fiddian-Green, R. G., R. C. Russell, and M. Hobsley. "Secretion-Induced Pyloric Reflux: Verification of the Mathematical Formula for Eliminating Reflux in Gastric Aspirate." *Brit. J. Surg.* 59 (1972): 903.

20. Hobsley, M. "Pyloric Reflux: A Modification of the Two-Component Hypothesis of Gastric Secretion." *Clinical Science and Molecular Medicine* 47 (1974): 131–141.

21. Faber, R. G., R. C. Russell, J. V. Parkin, P. Whitfield, and M. Hobsley. "Duodenal Reflux during Insulin-Stimulated Secretion." *Gut* 15 (1974): 880–884.

22. Faber, R. G., R. C. Russell, J. V. Parkin, P. Whitfield, and M. Hobsley. "The Predictive Accuracy of the Postvagotomy Insulin Test: A New Interpretation." *Gut*, 1975a: 337–342.

23. Burge, H., and J. R. Vane. "Method of Testing for Complete Nerve Section during Vagotomy." *British Med. J.* 1 (1958): 615–618.

24. Cox, A. J. "Stomach Size and Its Relation to Chronic Peptic Ulcer." *Arch. Path.* 54 (1952): 407.
25. Baron, J. H. "Peptic Ulcer, Gastric Secretion and Body Build." *Gut* 5 (1964): 83–85.
26. Baron, J. H. "Lean Body Mass, Gastric Acid and Peptic Ulcer." *Gut* (1969): 637–642.
27. Hassan, M. A., and M. Hobsley. "The Accurate Assessment of Maximal Gastric Secretion in Control Subjects and Patients with Duodenal Ulcer." *Brit. Med. J.* 1 (1971): 458–460.
28. Kronborg, O., J. Malmstrom, and P. M. Christiansen. "The Results of Truncal and Selective Vagotomy in Patients with Duodenal Ulcer." *Scand. J.* Gastroent. 5 (1970): 519–524.
29. Spencer, J., G. P. Burns, L. F. Y. Cheng, A. G. Cox, and R. B. Welbourn. "Difference between Males and Females in the Hollander Insulin Test." *Gut* 10 (1969): 307–310.
30. Emas, S., and I. Borg. "The Insulin Test: Negative and Positive Tests versus Numerical Values." *Scand. J. Gastroent.* 10(1975): 609–616.
31. Maybury, N. K., Faber, R.G., and Hobsley, M. "Postvagotomy Insulin Test: Improved Predictability of Ulcer Recurrence after Correction for Height and Collection Errors." *Gut* 18 (1977): 449–456.
32. Maybury, N. K., Russell, R.C.G., Faber, R.G., and Hobsley, M. "A New Interpretation of the Insulin Test Validated and then Compared with the Burge Test." *British Journal of Surgery* 64 (1977): 673–676.

CHAPTER 8:

Lecturer in Surgery, University of Leicester, 1977–1980

The day I started at the Leicester Royal Infirmary as lecturer in surgery, effectively as Professor Peter Bell's senior registrar, I was a little nervous. I had done no operating for the previous two years while working for my doctorate (DM), and on my first day I was thrown in at the deep end. To my relief and delight I found that all the skills of diagnosis and operating came back into play immediately.

Peter Bell was the inaugural professor of surgery at the new medical school in Leicester. He was a general surgeon with a special interest in vascular surgery and came down from Glasgow, where it was rumoured he had turned down a prestigious appointment to work in Leicester. He was later knighted for his services to surgery.

It was from Professor Bell that I learned diagnosis and vascular surgical technique and, of greater importance, when *not* to operate. He often said, "Being able to do an operation is not a reason for doing it." The operating suite at Leicester was vast, with seventeen operating theatres, alive with activity and a staff of about one hundred and fifty, but was more impersonal than the six at the Middlesex, or the two at Warwick hospitals where everyone knew everybody else.

One day every week, the professor had two operating theatres for the whole day. The day before, all the patients were admitted during the morning, and the professor did a "grand ward round" in the afternoon. Every patient was clerked by the houseman and one of the students, and presented to all those attending the round. We examined each patient in turn, looked at any X-rays, and discussed the diagnosis, management, and operation for the following day. Thus all the patients for an operation the next day were seen and everybody on the firm knew who they were. Of greater importance, everybody knew what operation they were to have and patients were marked with an indelible pen for side and site of their operation as described elsewhere.

The operating sessions were always interesting and rewarding to all the surgical staff and started at exactly nine in the morning. The patient in each theatre had been anaesthetised by a team of two anaesthetists, who had started a little earlier. In one theatre the professor and registrar (Reg) operated, and in the adjacent theatre the lecturer/senior registrar (SR) and senior house officer (SHO) operated. The lists ran all day, without stopping even for lunch. With the professor's method of running the theatres, there were always operations in progress in both theatres. Every member of the surgical team operated during the day commesurate with their experience. Each surgeon took a short break for lunch on an informal basis when an opportunity arose, while the remaining surgeon continued operating under indirect supervision; the same framework applied to the anaesthetists.

For example, in the first theatre, usually the day would start with a major vascular case, an aortic aneurysm to be replaced or an aorto-iliac bypass graft to be inserted. The registrar would open the abdomen with a long incision to expose the aorta and then assist the professor. Meanwhile, in the second theatre, a cholecystectomy might be the first operation of the day. The SHO would open the abdomen under the SR's supervision, and if the operation was straightforward the SHO would complete the removal of the gall-bladder with the SR as assistant. The SR would then go to the first theatre and join the professor in operating on the vascular case—initially assisting, but gradually in the weeks and months ahead, doing more and more of the operating. Meanwhile, the registrar would join the SHO in the second theatre and either operate himself or supervise the SHO in carrying out the second operation of the day. The level of operating was calibrated to the experience of each of the professor's assistants. The SHO might then assist the professor in a vagotomy and pyloroplasty carried out on a patient with a debilitating duodenal ulcer. Meanwhile, the SR would take the registrar through a colectomy for cancer of the colon. If an operation was proving difficult in the second theatre, then either the SR or the professor would go through to help, either by supervising or operating as appropriate. Which of us went would be the professor's decision. If he thought I, as the SR, was ready to continue on a vascular case solo, he would leave me to proceed and go to the other theatre to help. If not, I would go through.

So we would proceed until the early evening. It was fantastic for training and for the patients. The three junior surgeons would do a substantial amount of operating every day, and all felt very happy to be progressing in the art and science of surgery with every operation. The patients were well served, as the professor or SR was always available to immediately step in if an operation was difficult and before any problems had occurred. The professor was happy that a huge service work-load was achieved with every list. The juniors were happy that they could observe and learn the manoeuvres required to bring technically difficult operations to a successful close. The whole day was an excellent demonstration of teamwork.

This was also a brilliant way of economically using theatres to provide a first class service to the patients and hands-on learning for all the surgical staff, demonstrating apprenticeship in action. I copied and used this system for many years as a consultant until it was brought to an end in 2000 under one of the many reorganisations inflicted on the health service.

Leicester University had been the first new medical school in twenty years. The failure to build more medical schools over many decades was short sighted of all governments since the inception of the NHS in 1949. By 2012, this shortfall had resulted in one third of the doctors in the NHS having being born and trained overseas. This third, numbering eighty-eight thousand doctors, provide services that are invaluable, and without which the NHS would not function. The numbers of medical schools and places in British medical schools are not and never have been adequate to make Britain self-sufficient in doctors.

Shortly after I joined the staff at Leicester Royal Infirmary, the very first students were admitted for clinical training. There was great enthusiasm and eager anticipation amongst staff and students alike to get the new medical school started. Patients referred to the Leicester University Hospitals came from a large portion of Leicestershire, serving a population of about a million people. The effect was that the duty surgical firm could expect to admit up to thirty and sometimes more emergency patients during their take of twenty-four hours. Therefore, emergency operations were in progress a lot of the day and night as necessary. This provided an unparalleled and rich experience for the junior surgeons who would, as in Warwick, continue with the next day's planned work, however busy they had been,—a system I knew well and much enjoyed. I was also pleased to find that the general surgical firms at Leicester looked after all the head injuries, and I was once more involved in emergency neurosurgery.

One afternoon I received an urgent message from Alan Hamilton, my surgical registrar, to come to casualty immediately, as there was an unconscious baby in urgent need of attention. The baby had fallen out of his pram and onto his head an hour before. He had not been knocked unconscious by his fall and had screamed immediately, but had gradually become drowsy and difficult to rouse with the tell-tale sign of the pupil of the left eye dilating. The speed with which these events occurred meant that this child was suffering from an extradural haemorrhage due to the rupture of the temporal artery within the skull. The haematoma, or blood clot, was now pressing on the brain and beginning to render the child unconscious, and this pressure was causing the dilatation of his pupil. There was no time to waste. I rapidly explained the gravity of the situation to the baby's mother, leaving the SHO to obtain a signed consent to operate and then join us in theatre. Alan Hamilton carefully carried the baby to the theatre suite, while I ran ahead to clear an operating theatre.

The first operating theatre in the operating suite was set for a gynaecological operation. The patient was already anaesthetised and about to be wheeled from the anaesthetic room to the theatre. Very quickly I asked the anaesthetist to wheel his patient back to the anaesthetic room where she was reattached to the ventilator. There was just time to ask the gowned scrub nurse to open a craniotomy pack, where all the instruments were ready, presterilised, with everything needed to operate on this eighteen-month-old baby who was by now in a very serious state and completely unconscious.

The consultant anaesthetist who had so obligingly taken his patient back to the anaesthetic room was by chance also specialised in anaesthetics for babies and small children, and what is more, he had an assistant who could look after the displaced patient. With calmness and speed, the anaesthetist put up a drip and secured the baby for ventilation with a fine endotracheal tube. At this stage no anaesthetic was needed as the child was deeply unconscious. While this was being done, Alan and I rapidly scrubbed and gowned up. The patient had been draped by the scrub nurse.

A small incision into the scalp was made, and bleeding from the scalp edge was stopped with a retractor, so exposing the skull. All the experience I had gained at Warwick was put to use. With brace and bit, I cautiously drilled and removed a disc from the skull. To my delight the bleeding artery was immediately revealed; it lay on a substantial blood clot pressing on the brain. The bleeding artery was easily clipped above and below the tear from which the blood had been gushing. The blood clot was then sucked out. At this point the child moved and began to regain consciousness. Our anaesthetist gave our small patient a light anaesthetic. The wound was closed with a tiny drain in place to collect any oozing and the head was bandaged.

It is one of the greatest pleasures in life to give a child's mother the good news after her baby's brush with death. This baby went on to make a complete and uneventful recovery.

Some months later another notable emergency occurred. My car had broken down a few days earlier, and I had been offered a hearse by one of my wife's cousins as a temporary replacement. This vehicle was an ancient Austin Princess. On the night of the emergency in question, I was called from home by Alan Hamilton, who was with a patient in the casualty department at the Royal Infirmary. He said there was a man in the resuscitation room who had been stabbed in the left side of the chest. The blade had penetrated his heart causing a cardiac tamponade, where blood was pumping out of the heart through the stab wound, filling the space between the outer wall of the heart and the pericardium. As this space filled, the pressure built up, leaving less and less room for the normal flow of blood from the atrium to the ventricle, both of which were becoming compressed, significantly reducing the pumping of blood round the body. Cardiac arrest and death would rapidly follow if this was untreated.

Having correctly made the diagnosis of cardiac tamponade entirely on clinical grounds, Alan had plunged a large needle attached to a syringe under the ribs and into the space between the heart and the pericardium. He had successfully withdrawn blood, which gave the wounded man's heart enough room to keep beating for him to stay alive. At this point, Alan rang to inform me of the situation. I gave instructions for a theatre to be prepared, with notification to the resident anaesthetist to attend immediately. A sterile thoracotomy set was to be made ready while I raced to the hospital in the hearse. There was no time to go to the car park, so I left the vehicle outside casualty and went straight to theatre.

The wounded man was brought to the operating theatre at the same time as I arrived. Alan was still aspirating blood from the pericardium and successfully keeping the patient alive. The operation rapidly followed. I opened the left side of the chest, retracted the lung, and then widely opened the pericardium, which had a large clot of blood in it. The clot was removed, and the stab wound in the left ventricle, spurting blood with every heartbeat, was visible. Like the Dutch boy with his finger in the hole in the dyke, Alan Hamilton stopped any further loss of blood with a finger in the stab wound. Meanwhile, the anaesthetist restored the patient's blood volume with intravenous fluids and blood, and the scrub nurse prepared the sutures to close the wound in the heart. This was rapidly accomplished, and the bleeding stopped. I placed a drain in the pericardium, and closed the chest. The patient was taken to the intensive care unit. I then congratulated Alan on his brilliant performance, and I have to confess that I felt pretty pleased, too.

It did not surprise me when the next day the thoracic surgeon, Mr Bolton-Carter, who had taught me a great deal, summoned me to see him. I was thinking that he wanted to congratulate me on the previous night's operation. However, all he said was: "Ah, there you are, Maybury. There was a hearse parked outside casualty last night. Was it yours?" Slightly cautiously I answered in the affirmative, and he continued, "You shouldn't back two horses at once." That was it. I was dismissed, and the day's work continued as normal.

Back to the commonplace, the type of hernia repair being used in 1978 was the Maloney darn. The technique had been published in 1943 using a braided nylon suture to reinforce the posterior wall of the inguinal canal in an attempt to prevent a recurrent hernia from developing in the same place. This was a great advance on one pre-World War II technique of using floss silk in the hope that the intense scarring promoted by the inflammation caused by the silk would somehow do the job of reinforcing the inguinal canal. There were frequent infections, and the only way to cure these was to remove all the silk, which could harbour millions of pathogenic bacteria within its strands. These infections were often impossible to eradicate by oral or even intravenous antibiotics, because the silk was walled off from the bloodstream, and the bacteria lurked amongst the fibres of the silk. There were also infections in the braided nylon used in Maloney's darn, but this was much easier to find and remove on re-exploration than silk, as the nylon tended to break more slowly into fragments than the silk. Thus silk, which had been used as the suture material of choice for eighty years, from the time of Billroth in the 1880s, was finally being abandoned in the fifties and was obsolete by the sixties.

The other complication of these hernia repairs was that the recurrence rate was 5% in the first year after operation, and then another 10% occurred over the next ten years. It was true that 85% of hernias were successfully treated, but a 15% recurrence rate was too high, especially as it was known that a technique developed by a Canadian surgeon, Dr Edward Shouldice[1], in the post-war years, had developed a technique for hernia repair using braided wire with a recurrence rate of one in a thousand. This was excellent, even though Shouldice never accepted a patient for operation who presented as an emergency, such as a strangulated hernia. Patients suffering with these problems were always sent to the local general hospital. The only surgeon I knew who was an expert in this complex technique was Mr Brendan Devlin, with whom I had worked at St Thomas's Hospital, where I was a houseman, and he was the senior registrar on the firm.

In 1969, Brendan Devlin[2] arranged for two patients to be admitted every Saturday morning for repair of their inguinal hernias, which he accomplished that same morning using Shouldice's technique. These patients were discharged the next day, which was Sunday, so their presence did not block any beds for those patients being admitted on the Sunday for the Monday lists. Unfortunately I was too junior in my surgical career to learn this useful technique from him. These operations show what good results could be achieved using this technique. For Brendan this work would advance his career by publishing the results. This technique seemed a difficult procedure, as it was never widely used in the United Kingdom. However, the Shouldice Clinic was a success, and perhaps it was the first time a hospital and surgeons were dedicated to a single operation, and may mark the beginning of super-subspecialisation.

Vascular surgery technology and technique had advanced considerably on a broad front in the years since I had first been exposed to it at Warwick. The new synthetic grafts of woven Dacron were superior and easy to sew compared to the homographs from cadavers. As these new grafts were porous, it was necessary to prevent blood loss through the wall of the graft when they were sewn into place and the clamps released. To avoid this, they are sealed at the beginning of the operation with non-anticoagulated blood taken directly from the aorta at the very beginning of the operation.

Anaesthesia had improved and was safe. Intensive postoperative care was available, with resident anaesthetists present and on duty twenty-four hours a day. Fluid balance had improved, and intravenous nutrition was now available in ready prepared sterile packs suitable for attaching to a drip. Last, and of great importance, there was no longer any attempt to resect, or cut out, the whole aneurysm itself.

At operation, after the aorta had been secured above and below the aneurysm, it was now simply opened and any clot evacuated.

The graft is then laid within the aorta and sutured to the normal-size aorta above and below. The technique of these operations I learned from Professor Bell, first by assisting him, then carrying out parts of the operation under his direct supervision, and finally performing whole operations solo, with the professor available to advise or assist as necessary.

In practice it took me about eighteen months of assessing patients with vascular disease—as outpatients and when operating on them on a weekly basis—to learn how to carry out these difficult procedures, which on average now took one to two hours to carry out.

Of equal importance, as has already been mentioned, I learned the wisdom of not operating, unless an operation would be of benefit to the patient. In the case of claudication in a leg, perhaps it was not yet necessary, or perhaps the patient's limb was beyond salvage, and an operation would fail. In such a case, only an amputation would relieve the pain, provided the patient accepted this difficult and traumatic decision. I was gaining more experience and knowledge and would be soon ready to apply for a consultant post, confident that I could handle all the problems that would be sent to me.

One day when in the doctors' dining room in the Royal Infirmary, I overheard in a conversation that a consultant surgeon from Warwick had been admitted to the intensive care unit (ICU). I immediately went to see him. It was my old chief Mr John Marsh from Warwick, who was obviously very ill. I greeted him, and Mr Marsh responded with a look of recognition in his eyes. I noted that the X-ray viewing box at the bottom of his bed was visible to him. The whole left lung field was opaque, indicating severe malfunction on that side. The full sight of his own chest X-ray was pretty disturbing for the poor man, who had spent a lifetime looking at X-rays, so I took it down and filed it.

Mr Marsh had come to Leicester to pick up a new car. As he was driving it away, he suddenly felt a terrible pain between his upper abdomen and behind his xiphysternum, radiating through to his back. He parked his car, locked it, and walked the two hundred yards or so to the casualty of the Royal Infirmary. He walked right up to a casualty officer just inside the entrance and said, "I am in terrible pain; either I've perforated a duodenal ulcer, or I've had a myocardial infarct."

He then collapsed to the floor in front of the young doctor, who immediately diagnosed a cardiac arrest. After calling for assistance, he started resuscitation. Between John Marsh's prescience in getting himself to the hospital and collapsing at the feet of a doctor within yards of a fully equipped resuscitation room, he had placed himself in the best place possible to be revived without delay and it was to the credit of the casualty officer that Mr Marsh was successfully resuscitated and then moved to the ICU. He had no recollection of anything that had happened to him, although he did remember that he had come to Leicester to fetch a new car. I had a chat to Mrs Marsh when she visited, and although it was touch and go for a while, he survived and returned to work in due course. John March was a charming man from whom I had learned so much, and I was very pleased to watch him make a successful recovery.

I had started looking for a consultant post in the autumn of 1979. I had been a lecturer/senior registrar at Leicester for two and a half years. I had decided not to stay in academic surgery following an experience I had.

The Royal Infirmary had a huge new academic block with many splendid facilities including comfortable seminar rooms with armchairs. One afternoon I was taking a small group of first-year students and woke up to hear a voice droning in the background. I realised that I was dropping off to sleep and it was my own voice I could hear droning! This was in such contrast to a series of lectures

I had given in the university school of anatomy, "The Anatomy of Access for Operations in General Surgery." The lectures were well received and attended by all the staff as well as the students. For some reason, as a result of this contrast, accentuated by the fact that I had been so busy clinically that my research was no further advanced, that I felt I would be better working in a district general hospital. There, only clinical students would be attached to my firm. I was enthusiastic about teaching clinical surgery, while for some reason I did not have the same enthusiasm for the first-year students' syllabus.

It was time to have my own show. Most consultant surgeons were about forty years old before being appointed and there was some scepticism that at thirty-six, and with such a short time as a lecturer/senior registrar, I could succeed. Even so the search for jobs began. There were no openings in Leicester, even though there was a track record of appointing their own trainees to consultant posts so I needed to look further afield.

1. Dr Edward Earle Shouldice, (1932–1965). Developed a natural-tissue, tension-free hernia repair during WWII and opened a clinic specialising in hernia repairs in 1945.

2. Devlin, H. Brendan, & Kingsnorth, Andrew. Management of Abdominal Hernias. Second Edition. 1988. Publisher, Chapman & Hall Medical, London.

CHAPTER 9

Consultant General Surgeon, Wigan and Leigh NHS Trust, 1980–2001

a. Introduction and administration
b. Vascular surgery,—the development of a vascular surgical service
c. Vascular surgery,—graft infection and prophylactic antibiotics
d. Trauma surgery and its decline.
e. Biliary surgery,—obstructive jaundice before and after the development of endoscopic operative techniques
f. Biliary surgery,—cholecystectomy, the change from open to laparoscopic operations
g. Gut surgery,—the oesophagus
h. Gut surgery,—screening for colonic cancer
i. Gut surgery,—gastric surgery and surgery for duodenal ulcers
j. Audit of inguinal hernia repair
k. Training surgical registrars
l. Registrar appointments
m. Training of registrars and the European Working Time Directive, EWTD1998
n. The grand round and its demise
o. Finances
p. References

a. Introduction and administration

An advertisement in the *British Medical Journal* seeking a general surgeon for Wigan was seen. Initially I was not inclined to apply. My wife told me that Wigan was an ancient town called Coccium in Roman times, and on this slim recommendation, we went to visit Wigan's Royal Albert Edward Infirmary. It was a Victorian foundation, opened in 1873, coincidentally with the dawn of the golden age of general surgery, by Albert Edward the Prince of Wales. In 1979, much of the original hospital was still in use, but there were also a lot of temporary wooden buildings from World War II that now served for outpatients and some wards. The atmosphere in the hospital was good and I was not put off by a Manchester surgeon telling me that general surgery at Wigan was for "hernia and varicose vein merchants." Everyone I met was very friendly, and on talking to staff, it was apparent that no oesophageal or peripheral vascular surgery was carried out there. Perhaps Wigan was just the challenge that I was looking for.

On a further visit before the interview, I walked through the original Victorian entrance to the Royal Albert Edward Infirmary (RAEI). Thinking that the hospital was probably due for a rebuild, brought to mind some advice Mr John Marsh had given me. "Metaphorically speaking, when you are being interviewed for a consultant post, they will tell you that the pile of bricks you see in the corner is going to be a new hospital. Don't believe them." At Warwick, before Mr Marsh was appointed as a consultant surgeon, he was told that a new hospital was about to be built. The new hospital was built—but not until after he had retired. With these words in mind, I looked into the World War II wooden huts that were used as the surgical outpatients department and concluded they could serve for a few more decades. The staff I met, who included Sister Barbara Siney of Swinley surgical ward, were all very welcoming and pleasant. I also took the opportunity to speak with the sister in charge of the twin operating theatres, built on the same model as the old Victorian theatres at St

Thomas's Hospital, which were open to each other. I asked her what instruments there were for vascular surgery, only to be informed that there weren't any, nor were there any for oesophageal surgery. This confirmed that Wigan was a place to be to introduce new specialities and techniques, so I applied for the consultant general surgeon's post. At interview, the chairman of the regional health authority, Mr Sidney Hamburger, famously said, "If you can't work in Wigan, you can't work anywhere!"

I was appointed and felt this was a great opportunity to make a difference to help improve the surgical services in the area. So I gave in my notice at Leicester and began to prepare to start in Wigan on All Fools Day, 1980!

On the appointed day, I arrived with eager anticipation and immediately went to the surgical wards to see my first patients, who had been selected and admitted by my predecessor, Mr Weatherstone-Wilson, for operations that morning. He had kindly arranged this, as waiting lists were long, and no list was to be wasted, even on my first day. Having seen all the patients and found everything satisfactory, I spent the morning operating. Everything went without a hitch. It was action immediately from day one with no induction process or formal introductions to colleagues.

In the early days, contact with colleagues of all specialities was easy, because there was a doctors' dining room, where I lunched whenever possible, to meet and talk shop with colleagues. It was because of the dining room, while it existed, that no formal induction for new consultants was really needed, as one quickly met most of one's colleagues of all specialities. It was a good place to discuss patients with difficult problems and to seek advice. As soon as we had finished eating, one or two colleagues and I would gather our junior staff, who also ate there, to visit the ward to see a patient who had been discussed over lunch and continue our deliberations. This provided not only a first-class service to patients but also good experience for my junior staff. Unfortunately, in the mid-eighties the doctors' dining room was closed on grounds of egalitarianism and anti-elitism, a very retrograde step from a clinical point of view. Consultants were told they could use the general canteen, which was well equipped (and the food was better), but because it was also used by all the non-medical staff and some mobile patients and relatives, it was now impossible to talk in detail about patients and be sure of confidentiality, and so the consultants never used the general canteen. The informal and informative discussions over lunch ceased, and the consultants became increasingly isolated clinically.

Fifteen years later, when I had been elected as chairman of the staff committee, a questionnaire was sent to seek the views of my colleagues concerning the possibility of a doctors' dining room. If re-established, would it be patronised? The response was a surprise, because most colleagues were doing what I did at lunch-time, which was to continue to work. Only one consultant went to a local pub, possibly to grab a sandwich. The majority decided that if there was a doctors' dining room they would not use it, which was a pity; so the matter was dropped.

My first operating list was followed by a complete ward round with Mr Paul Chui, my registrar, who proved to be an experienced and competent surgeon. There were four lists a week allocated to me at the RAEI. Every Thursday there were three half days allocated, with all-day operating in one theatre and a twin list in the adjacent theatre during the morning. The fourth list was on Friday morning. The twin lists on Thursday mornings were invaluable for teaching, and at the same time, providing an excellent service to the local people. Later that first day, I drove seven miles to Leigh Infirmary, where I was met by the surgical registrar, Mr Bhatnager. He confirmed that one list a week was scheduled for me every Friday morning in the Leigh Infirmary operating theatre. This was not ideal, as I also had the operating list at the same time at the RAEI. This arrangement was the cause of some anxiety. However, with Mr Bhatnager in Leigh Infirmary and Mr Chui at the Royal Albert

Edward Infirmary, coupled with taking great care in the selection of patients to be operated on in the hospital I was not attending, there were no untoward operative or postoperative complications caused by lack of supervision. This, of course, spoke well of the registrars concerned, who felt that they had ownership and responsibility for continuity of care. Fortunately, like Mr Chui at Wigan, Mr Bhatnager was a very experienced surgeon. On completing my round at Leigh Infirmary, I drove to Billinge Hospital, the third of the hospitals in which I had been allocated beds. Billinge Hospital was seventeen miles away towards St Helens. This hospital was largely concerned with obstetrics and gynaecology, psychiatry, and surgery. General surgery was allotted one ward with four operating lists every week of which one, on Tuesday afternoons, was mine.

After completing the first tour of my new domain, the problems that I had inherited gradually began to sink in. With patients in all three hospitals of the Wigan and Leigh Health Authority, it meant almost daily trips between the hospitals for ward rounds, operating lists, and clinics. Not surprisingly, during the first few years of working in Wigan I drove thousands of miles between the hospitals each year. This consumed the equivalent of almost a whole day a week in travelling, which was of course a waste of time.

My determination from day one was that I would consolidate my practice into one hospital as soon as possible. Since most of my inpatients were in the RAEI, and this was where the intensive care unit for the hospital group was situated, it was the obvious choice. This would not only save the time taken up in driving, but also it would also enable me to keep a close eye on all my patients and be a much better arrangement for the junior staff.

There were four consultant surgeons at Wigan, each with their own firm. The allocation of surgical beds was unusual, compared to my previous experience. All the general surgical beds in five wards throughout the health authority's hospitals were held in common, to be used as needed by the surgeons—an arrangement that worked well and in many ways was very much to my advantage, as I tended to have more inpatients than my colleagues and could therefore use more beds for my patients. My firm consisted of me, the only consultant, two registrars, one at the RAEI working solely for me, and the other at Leigh Infirmary who worked for all four consultants. I had two senior house officers, one each at Wigan and Leigh, and three house officers, one at each at the three hospitals.

Two of the house officer posts were unsatisfactory. In Leigh, the house officer was shared by two consultants and would receive training in theatre two half days a week, which did not offer adequate experience of the surgical conditions of patients admitted for surgery. There was an accident and emergency department (A&E) at Leigh Infirmary that was open twenty-four hours a day, giving an opportunity to see and admit trauma cases. Billinge Hospital was the worst possible posting for a house officer, who worked for all four consultants; this was unsatisfactory. There were four operating lists weekly, each with a different consultant, no A&E, so no emergencies to see or gain experience from, and there was no registrar. That the house officer would work alone most of the time was also unsafe and unacceptable.

I had no idea in April 1980 that it would take three years to close the surgical ward at Billinge Hospital and concentrate the general surgical presence in Wigan, or that it would take even longer to withdraw from Leigh Infirmary. I was in the RAEI every day and also carried out ward rounds twice a week in each of the other hospitals. Every Saturday morning I always did a complete ward round in all three hospitals to check to see if there were any problems from the week's operating and, if so, sort them out. Then there were urgent domiciliary visits requested by GPs. It was usually late afternoon before I returned home, but these domiciliary visits were often clinically very valuable. Many of these patients were seriously ill, and seeing a consultant would reassure the patient and relatives, as well as the GP, that further treatment had been considered, and appropriate arrangements could then be made for admission for those in need of surgery. Those for whom hospital had nothing further to offer would be saved the upheaval of admission and would be reassured and made comfortable at home.

Late in my second year at Wigan I was elected to be chairman of the division of general surgery. This enabled me to talk regularly with my colleague who represented the division of gynaecology and obstetrics. Being chairman of a division sounds very grand, but in reality it's only an example of "Buggin's turn." All NHS consultants were equal in both fact and pay. Each speciality group had to elect from amongst themselves someone to represent the group on the medical executive committee (MEC) of that time. This committee made recommendations to the area health authority concerning all aspects of management of the hospital, and these recommendations were often accepted. The direct control of the finances had passed out of the hands of the medical profession in 1974. However, the composition of the board of the area health authority had not altered much, being comprised of a general manager, the finance officer, several lay appointees, two working consultants, and the matron. The direct power of the consultants had gone, but strong influence still remained in the governing body in the early eighties.

The medical executive committee met fortnightly, and many divisions appointed their newest member as chairman of their division. The whole assemblage was designated the "cogwheel" system. Meeting regularly as a member of this committee, I gradually persuaded Miss Betty Hargreaves from the gynaecological division of the benefits of swapping wards. This was eventually agreed. As a result, I stopped working at Billinge Hospital, and no more house officers suffered in this inadequate post.

The cogwheel system did not last long. It was abolished with the appointment of a chief executive on a salary not only greater than that of the former administrator but also greater than the consultants. This change was accompanied by a new major overhaul of the facilities of the newly named Wigan and Leigh NHS Trust.

The new trust board had only one consultant, who was appointed by the regional health authority and not elected by colleagues. This person was not a representative and was fairly powerless, being heavily outnumbered by an increase of lay members and administrators, including a human resources officer. One of the first jobs for the trust was to reduce the bed numbers by fifty percent. This was accomplished in the acute sector by closure of convalescent hospitals and hospital wards. It was even worse and disproportionate for the psychiatrists, with the closure of all the large psychiatric hospitals and the start of "care in the community," which has had a significant impact on society as a whole, but that is a different story. These changes saw a huge shift in the way patients were managed as they passed through the hospital, and this is described later.

On the administrative side, there was a full-time secretary attached to my firm who worked for me. Mrs Gillian Bennett was an excellent medical secretary. She was cheerful, well organised, remembered everybody's name, especially the patients, and everything the firm was doing. Essentially a PA, although not paid as such, she was adept at helping junior staff, especially the women with any problems they might have. Gillian ran the administration of the firm and came to every outpatient clinic, which always overran the time allocated to it, as any patient about whom a GP was concerned was sent up immediately to be seen. Throughout the outpatient session, I dictated as I went along. Five minutes after the last patient was seen the letters from the clinic were already typed, without error, and ready to sign. They were posted that day, a remarkable service. The office she worked from was hers as consultants did not have offices in the eighties.

In 1980 there was very little diagnostic equipment at the RAEI. The X-ray department was staffed by two consultant radiologists. Dr Norman Crosby worked endlessly and carried out contrast X-rays of the GI tract, kidneys, gall-bladder, and arteries. He wielded the single and almost-defunct upper-gastro-intestinal endoscope in the hospital, which was useful in diagnosing gastric cancers and duodenal ulcers, but nothing much else, due to its broken fibre-optic filaments, and it did not have a channel for taking biopsies. Haematology and biochemistry had been in place for some years, and of course the consultant histopathologists were busy. The most basic and important diagnostic skills in surgery remained the detailed history and clinical examination of the patient.

b. Vascular surgery,—the development of a vascular surgical service

Having recently worked for Professor Bell, it seemed proper that all the vascular cases, both elective and emergency, should come under my care, especially as none of my colleagues were trained in this branch of surgery. My aim was to provide a consistent service over the next few years until another general surgeon with an interest in vascular surgery could be appointed. So for several years I worked in this endeavour alone. Before taking up my post at Wigan, and by arrangement with the theatre sister, one new vascular instrument was bought every week from the small surgical instrument budget allocated to each new surgeon. These purchases started during the three months before my arrival. The instruments bought were chosen for their quality and purpose, care being taken that they did not duplicate the instruments that the theatre superintendent at Leicester Royal Infirmary had kindly promised she could spare me from surplus stock. This was very pleasing, as it meant that when I started to work at Wigan, I would have one complete set of vascular instruments available, enabling me to carry out vascular operations, including aortic surgery, both elective and emergency.

This one set of vascular instruments was adequate at RAEI, because in 1980 all surgical instruments were cleaned and autoclaved in the theatre suite by the nursing staff. So by deliberately not listing two vascular cases consecutively on an operating list, a single set of vascular instruments would be sufficient to provide a vascular service, as there would be time for these precious instruments to be cleaned and autoclaved during the intervening non-vascular operation.

As a member of the Vascular Surgical Society (VSS), which had carried out a national survey, I was aware that there were at least thirty to forty patients every year in Wigan who were not receiving the vascular operations that they needed, had the facilities been available. This was the calculation of potential work-load that I thought could be accommodated by the hospital and my firm. Business plans had not been heard of in those days, nor indeed were they asked for. The VSS's survey proved to be accurate, and in the course of time, due to the aging of the population over the next twenty years, the volume of vascular operations increased substantially (chapter 10, table 10). Vascular surgery was very much in the remit of general surgeons. Eventually, in 2012, after my retirement, it was recognised as a speciality in its own right with surgeons dedicated exclusively to its practice.

In this way all vascular emergencies in the Wigan area came under my care, including leaking aortic aneurysms and cases of acute or critical limb ischaemia, either from vascular disease or trauma to the great arteries. Thus I found myself on call seven days a week for these emergencies. This was in addition to my routine on-call duties on the general surgical rota. This was reminiscent of my time in Warwick, but even more relentless. Wigan and Leigh Health Authority covered a large area, including not only the towns of Wigan and Leigh but also Astley, Ashton-in-Makerfield, Hindley, and many small villages with a total population of nearly four hundred thousand people. Many nights and weekends found me operating at the infirmary on vascular and other emergencies.

Being on call permanently lasted four years, until two new consultants, Mr John Mosley and Mr Malcolm Holbrook, were appointed in quick succession to work full time at Leigh Infirmary and share in the vascular admissions rota. Leigh Infirmary was, at the time of their appointment, designated to be a district general hospital (DGH) in its own right. Unfortunately, this plan was dropped two years later and is an example of an NHS decision being reversed by another tier of its bureaucracy, this made planning very difficult. Fortunately, in spite of this, both my new colleagues continued to share in the burden of the vascular emergency rota and significantly reduced my emergency surgical burden. It also enabled me to withdraw from any work at Leigh Infirmary. The burden of being on call all the time before these new appointments were made would now be considered intolerable and unacceptable. It was hard work, but in the early 1980s I was determined to make Wigan and Leigh a respected centre for vascular surgery and in this way stop the automatic referral of vascular and upper gut surgery to Manchester.

The admission of vascular emergencies was a great opportunity to train staff, both medical and nursing, in the management of these difficult cases. When I was setting up the vascular unit, each and every vascular operation was discussed pre-, inter-, and postoperatively with medical and nursing staff. Following the operation I went with the patient to the ICU to supervise and teach the nurses how to look after the patients. I trained the nurses to notice when something was not quite right with the patient and not to ignore it but draw my attention to their concerns about the patient, day or night. In the early days, it was always necessary for me to go in to the infirmary whenever called. Occasionally it meant taking the patient back to theatre because of haemorrhage or an unexpected occlusion of a graft. These complications could usually be sorted out safely by prompt intervention. Delay could be literally fatal, and I impressed on them that that I did not want to see a patient's observation chart recording a patient's deteriorating condition before the telephone was picked up.

The staff learned quickly, and within a few months all was running smoothly, and I was no longer needed in the ICU so often. The skill and dedication of the nursing staff and consultant anaesthetists was very much appreciated. I principally worked with Dr Wyn Jones and Dr Venkataraman, always known as Dr Venkat. We were often working together late into the night to provide a good service by maintaining the stability of the patients postoperatively. It was always reassuring to be able to rely on my colleagues' great skill and that of other anaesthetists, amongst whom were Dr Pat Ford and Dr John Crook and many others.

One task that needed to be undertaken was the delicate matter of persuading my physician colleagues not to order arteriograms on patients they suspected of having peripheral arterial disease. Symptomatic peripheral arterial disease can usually be diagnosed from the history and clinical findings alone. A hand-held Doppler ultrasound, which became available at that time, could be helpful.

Arteriograms were and are not free from occasional—but very severe—complications and should only be used as a "road map" for an operation, when and only when a vascular surgeon decided that an operation was needed if the arteriograms showed that it was technically possible. In this case a contemporary arteriogram was needed, as last year's X-rays would be out of date.

Some vascular trauma patients still stand out in my mind. While I was operating at eleven o'clock one night in 1989, my SHO rang to say he had an unusual case in the A&E department. I asked him to come up to the theatre so he could tell me about it. It was a strange tale. Earlier, a man had been brought in to the A&E department with an upper arm injury. It transpired that the injured man was a zoo-keeper at the Wigan Municipal Zoo. A camel had leaned over a six-foot fence, grabbed him by the top of his left upper arm, and pulled him over the fence. He was rescued by a colleague.

He was taken to the A&E department complaining of pain with some loss of sensation in his arm. There were large puncture wounds over the deltoid and in his axilla. The SHO said he had found a radial pulse and on being asked if it was normal, replied that he could only identify it by using a Doppler ultrasound. I asked my SHO what he proposed doing; and he said he planned to bring the patient to theatre to clean the puncture wounds and sew them up. He explained that the puncture wounds, caused by the camel's molars, were large. The man had been given an antitetanus injection. I then asked that the patient be brought to the operating theatre following the operation I was then doing. The SHO asked why, and we discussed the patient's likely injuries.

The patient was six feet tall (188 cm) and weighed 12 stone (76 kg). This was the weight pulling on his upper arm as he was dragged over the fence. His loss of sensation was probably the result of the radial nerve being crushed against the humerus by the animal's teeth. The weak pulse at the wrist, in the absence of a generalised low blood pressure, indicated a significant injury to the axillary artery. The duty consultant radiologist was called, an emergency operative arteriogram then showed a total obstruction of the axillary artery. This I then repaired, using a reversed segment of the patient's own saphenous vein. Function of the radial nerve, which was not severed, recovered spontaneously over the next few months under the supervision of my orthopaedic colleague Mr Brian Livingstone. A camel injury thousands of miles from the desert caused some amusement. The municipal zoo was rightly closed sometime afterwards as not being of a sufficient standard for modern times.

There were two more cases of arterial trauma of especial note that involved rupture of the axillary artery. In both cases, in separate accidents, the casualties had been riding motorcycles. One had hit a tree with his left shoulder, and the other had hit a lamp-post, also with the left shoulder. I had learned the detailed practical anatomy of the axilla and how to safely operate within its complex anatomy while prosecting, and then later at the Middlesex Hospital while performing Patey's modified radical mastectomy that had superceded the now-obsolete Halstead's radical mastectomy.

One of the two motorcyclists was also a professional rugby league player, which added a new dimension of difficulty. The only professional rugger players in the eighties were those who played rugby league, a species of the game mainly played in the North of

England, and at which Wigan excelled. At that time these sports-men were far ahead in training and fitness compared to rugby union players, who were still amateur. The consequence of this fitness was the huge muscle bulk these sportsmen developed. When I operated on this super-fit man, it was his muscles that caused great prob-lems. Not only their bulk, but also their power was such that they were incredibly difficult to retract to gain access to the ruptured artery. This was so difficult that success was not certain. In addi-tion, where muscle needed to be divided, the resulting bleeding was so profuse due to its phenomenal vascularity that blood transfusion was required for this alone. Both men recovered after successful re-pair of their axillary arteries. Unfortunately the rugger player also had severely damaged his axillary plexus by stretching the nerves at the time of impact, and sadly, he never returned to the playing field.

While taking my first outpatient clinic at Leigh Infirmary, a tall, slim and, to me, old consultant came into the room and sat down on my desk. He introduced himself as Dr Bunt White, the consul-tant haematologist. I waited expectantly to hear what he had to say. "May I call you Keith?" I nodded, and he proceeded, "What we need here is an old-fashioned general surgeon"—he paused—"I hear that you intend to do vascular surgery." I nodded. "Pity," he said, "it's such a waste of blood." Since he was the doctor respon-sible for providing cross-matched blood when needed during such an operation, this statement took me aback, and I said something feeble, such as I would be careful. At this he took his leave.

Over the next few years I got to know Dr White well and appre-ciate his humour, skills, and help. I was eventually able to put his opening remarks to me into context. One of my colleagues, some time before my arrival in Wigan, had attempted two emergency vascular operations with considerable loss of blood, using thirty units (pints) in one case and only a little less in another. Vascular surgery now flourished without undue use of the transfusion ser-vice. By the early nineties there were five general surgeons in post, all carrying out emergency vascular surgery, also the volume of elective vascular surgery steadily increased, especially after the appointment to the staff of Mr John Mosley, an accomplished vascular surgeon who had been trained at the Middlesex Hospital.

c. Vascular surgery,—graft infection and prophylactic antibiotics

Every effort was made to avoid postoperative wound infection by using prophylactic antibiotics in addition to the aseptic technique. Prevention was the best way to avoid the catastrophic complications of infection in patients following insertion of synthetic vascular grafts. (See the case history of an infected graft in the appendix). In the early eighties, antibiotic prophylaxis consisted of a week's course, starting twenty-four hours before the operation. The antibiotic usually used was one of the penicillins. It is well known that inappropriate antibiotics, or low tissue levels of antibiotics, encourages the evolution of bacterial resistance.

Unfortunately, arterial graft infections almost always become chronic. Antibiotics cannot reach bacteria lodged in the interstices of the woven or knitted foreign materials from which grafts are made. Grafts are inert and cannot be vascularised, so antibiotics cannot be delivered at therapeutic doses to any pathological bacterial colonies. Diffusion is the only way for antibiotics to reach the graft, and then it's only at a very low concentration. Interestingly, this low concentration of antibiotic reaching the graft establishes an environment conducive to the evolution of antibiotic resistance. Since a subtherapeutic concentration of antibiotic does not kill all the target bacteria, then those few bacteria that have the slightest resistance to the antibiotic survive and reproduce. This same process brought floss silk into disrepute as a material used for hernia repair after the Second World War, as bacteria can secrete themselves, out of reach of antibiotics, amongst the fibres of the silk.

By the mideighties, the policy was to give a patient receiving a graft a single intravenous injection of a cephalosporin immediately after the anaesthetic and just before starting the operation. The principle was to ensure that the highest possible therapeutic level of antibiotic was circulating throughout the body at the beginning and during the operation. This would ensure that blood needed to seal an otherwise porous synthetic graft would have a high antibiotic level, and all tissues operated on and handled during the operation would already have a high level of antibiotic present. By this means, it was hoped that the chance of a graft infection taking place was reduced and the possibility of facilitating the evolution of resistant strains was also reduced.

The rationale for using prophylactic antibiotics was encouraged by evidence of their efficacy in preventing sepsis in a paper by Kaiser et al. from the Vanderbilt University School of Medicine titled "Antibiotic Prophylaxis in Vascular Surgery." It was presented at the annual meeting of the American Surgical Association in April 1978. In their clinical trial, comparison was made between a placebo and the antibiotic cefazolin as prophylaxis against infection in vascular operations, including surgery for aortic aneurysms.

Four hundred and sixty-two patients were studied between 1976 and 1977. The results were highly significant with an infection rate of 6.8% in the placebo group and 0.9% in the cephalosporin group. The trial looked mainly at the incidence of wound infection, but in the discussion it was noted that the occurrence of graft infections occurred in four patients in the placebo group, and two of them died as a result.

The appendix gives a case history of an aortic graft infection.

d. Trauma surgery and its decline.

Up until the mid-eighties, trauma patients continued to pour into the A&E department much as they had into casualty at Warwick Hospital ten years earlier. This volume of patients suffering serious trauma then gradually declined during the later eighties. At that time the only safe operation to save a patient who had a ruptured spleen was to carry out an emergency exploratory laparotomy, and if the spleen was bleeding, remove the whole organ. As a houseman when assisting my chief, Mr Nevin, during an operation at St Thomas's Hospital in 1969, the senior consultant physician, appeared in the elevated viewing gallery of the old theatres and called down to Mr Nevin. "Bob, you know I am interested in this patient. Could you take a biopsy of the spleen?" The response was immediate. "You can have it all or none." This tale illustrates the state of surgery on the spleen in 1969 and up to the mid eighties. Gradually surgical salvage of the spleen, or part of the spleen, was attempted and became increasingly successful in avoiding the long-term risk of infections in postsplenectomy patients.

This salvage operation made use of the knowledge that each segment of the spleen is served by an end artery. If one or more segments of the injured spleen have not been damaged, then these can be preserved by first removing all the damaged segments after ligating their arteries and veins. This approach to splenic preservation was assisted by using an absorbable material that dissolved over a few weeks. It acted like a net in which to wrap the functioning splenic remnant.

The confidence to attempt to salvage the spleen or part of the spleen was made feasible by improved technology in the definition of ultrasound imaging, combined with the skill of radiologists and radiographers in interpreting these images. By the nineties, a patient suspected of having a ruptured spleen would have the diagnosis rapidly confirmed by this means. Thus, a patient who was haemo-dynamically stable with a small splenic tear could now be monitored by serial ultrasound examinations. If a small blood clot or haematoma remained stable, then recovery without surgery was a possibility. However, if the haematoma increased rapidly, then exploratory laparotomy would become mandatory.

The same methodology was also used to monitor any minor postsplenectomy haemorrhage. If a haematoma became clinically large enough it could be drained percutaneously with a needle under ultrasound guidance, likewise avoiding a further operation. With these advances in technology and skill, considerable success was achieved in preserving some viable splenic tissue. The converse was true in carrying out elective splenectomies when requested by the haematologists, particularly in cases of thrombocytopaenic purpura (ch 10, table 10). In these cases, the skill lay not just in removing the spleen but also in searching out and removing any separate splenuncules, which, if not found, would slowly grow in size and cause a return of premature breakdown of red blood cells.

During the nineties, the admission of serious trauma into the A&E decreased significantly. This was good news for the population at large and had come about for many reasons, the chief being the regular use of seatbelts and the amazing increase in the volume of traffic forcing an overall reduction of speed on all roads including motorways.

TABLE 3A

Traffic Acidents.	1980	2000	2005	2012
Traffic in billions of miles.	150	275	-	-
Killed	5,935	3,409	-	1,754
Serious Injuries	58,000	38,000	-	23,039
Motorway death % total.	-	-	6.2%	-
Motorway serious injury % total.	-	-	3.3%	-

Table 3A *Traffic as measured in billions of miles driven rose significantly between 1980 and 2000. Paradoxically, the decline in road deaths was 57% and the serious injury numbers fell by 65% in the* *same 20 years. Most major injuries admitted to RAEI were motor-way accidents, and the figures for 2005 are given to illustrate how safe motorways are compared with urban areas from where most serious injuries emanate.*

Thus the volume of major trauma being admitted to RAEI over the years 1980–2000 was steadily reduced. By 2000, the opportunity for teaching the registrars the management and surgery of this aspect of what I should now call "old" general surgery was reduced due to the low numbers of seriously injured patients. In fact, the management and surgery of major trauma as an expected skill of the general surgeon in a large district general hospital had reduced significantly by 2000.

The data in table 3A supports the current suggestion (2013) to only have fully staffed A&D departments in the large conurbations of England. This, coupled with the significant reduction in time spent training the new generation of surgeons, means that to be fully staffed, a modern A&E should ideally be large, with a consultant staff of experienced surgeons in all relevant specialities on duty to manage a considerable daily throughput.

Unfortunately, the registrars received no training in emergency neurosurgery. On arriving in Wigan, I found that the orthopaedic surgeons admitted head injuries under their care. They carried out no emergency neurosurgery themselves and transferred all patients with suspected intracranial haemorrhage to the neurosurgical department in Manchester. I would have liked to take these patients under my care; however, my commitment to provide a vascular emergency surgery service with my other general surgery commitments meant that I could not take on another open-ended commitment.

So the status quo remained. I did continue to be concerned about the few patients with extradural haemorrhages, who can deteriorate rapidly.

e. Biliary surgery,—obstructive jaundice and its management before and after the development of endoscopic operative techniques

In the eighties, a blood test could usually differentiate between obstructive or infective causes of jaundice. If it was obstructive, then an urgent operation was indicated. A plain abdominal X-ray would show calcified gall-stones, indicating these as the probable cause of obstruction. However, if the plain X-ray showed nothing, then the jaundice might still be due to stones, as 90% of gall-stones are radiolucent. In these circumstances, an X-ray could not differentiate between gall-stones or cancer as the cause of the jaundice.

Therefore, patients with obstructive jaundice were offered an urgent laparotomy. This was the only way to make the diagnosis; untreated obstructive jaundice leads to liver failure. Those with stones were cured by this approach, as a cholecystectomy and exploration of the common bile duct with clearance of obstructing stones could be effected operatively. Those with cancer were usually inoperable due to advanced disease, although in some of these patients a short-to-moderate remission might be achieved if a bypass was possible. If a bypass was not technically possible, then the abdomen was closed, and the patient and relatives were informed of the hopeless prognosis.

Exploratory laparotomy for obstructive jaundice gradually became obsolete by the midnineties. Table 3 shows that this operation was quite common in the eighties and tailed off thereafter, to being a rare occurrence by 2000. This change was accomplished by the development of sophistocated endoscopes and a skilled endoscopist. The days of a surgeon using clinical skills with simple tests and surgery were drawing to a close.

In 1983, a new colleague, Dr Colin Bate, joined the staff at the RAEI as a consultant physician. Formerly of the Royal Army Medical Corps and an expert in thalassaemia, he recognised an opportunity to develop an endoscopy service and immediately set to work to persuade the health authority to buy endoscopes for the upper and lower gastro-intestinal tracts.

	TABLE 3									
A = General exploratory laparotomy										
B = Laparotomy for obstructive jaundice										
	1980	1981	1982	1983	1984	1985	1988	1990	1995	1999	2000
A	12	25	13	24	16	18	40	16	15	9	7
B	11	4	6	8	6	5	3	1	0	0	0

Table 3 is an extract from ch 10 table 10. Diagnostic laparotomies for obstructive jaundice were in decline by the late eighties due to the rise of therapeutic endoscopic intervention. The general exploratory laparotomies included patients whose symptoms warranted exploration and included patients with subacute obstruction or Crohn's disease, and a small group with radiation iliitis where small-bowel resections were necessary.

The skill of using an endoscope therapeutically was still novel, but by the late eighties, following advances in light technology and instrumentation, new techniques were developed, and patients with obstructive jaundice began to be referred to the new endoscopy department as their first port of call, rather than to the surgeon. It was now possible to identify and view endoscopically and insert a cannula into the opening of the common bile duct into the duodenum (papilla of Vater). Dye could then be injected, and X-rays taken to show pathology in the biliary tree and differentiate between biliary stones and cancer.

In the case of stones, the papilla of Vater could now be widely opened by an endoscopically performed sphincterotomy and the stones removed by snaring them in a collapsible wire basket. Removal of gall-stones from the CBD often avoided any necessity for open surgery because stones remaining in the gall-bladder are quite frequently asymptomatic. If the stones proved impossible to remove endoscopically, then a stent could be inserted past them, so enabling the bile to drain and the jaundice to settle, after which an elective operation would be arranged with the patient knowing the diagnosis.

If the X-rays of the CBD, taken following injection of dye down the endoscope, revealed a cancer, then an endoscopic biopsy was possible to confirm the diagnosis. At the same session, a stent could usually be pushed past the tumour into the dilated CBD above, enabling the bile to drain and the jaundice to settle. In the case of cancer, this manoeuvre bought time. There was time for the jaundice to settle once the pent-up bile was draining into the gut, time for the histological analysis of a biopsy specimen, and time to carry out further investigations such as computerised tomography (CT) or magnetic resonance imaging (MRI), when these became available in the nineties. There was also time for the patient to be informed of the diagnosis and for any options for further treatment to be discussed. This eliminating the uncertainty of the diagnosis or what was to be done. Before these options were available, a semi-emergency laparotomy was imperative to prevent liver failure.

Patients with jaundice caused by the uncommon papillary carcinoma, or a cancer restricted to the head of the pancreas, were candidates for a pancreatectomy (Whipple's operation). This could now be planned and carried out on a fit patient whose jaundice had resolved. Whipple's operation was a satisfying operation to perform. The anatomy is complex, and the operation is technically difficult. It was not a common operation and table 10 shows twelve such operations over the eleven years analysed. In this group, there was one perioperative death in a forty year old man who developed pneumonia and died a month postoperatively, his histology showed clinically undetectable widespread microscopic metastases. Two patients developed fistulae that healed spontaneously. One patient who underwent Whipple's operation belonged to a family with multiple endocrine neoplasia and is described in the appendix.

Open cholecystectomy was one of the staples of the work of a general surgeon. It was the operation par excellence that marked the progress of an SHO graduating from intermediate to major surgery. This operation, like all others, can be straightforward or very difficult, and in the latter case, it can, without great care, lead to damage to the common bile duct (CBD).

Sir Anthony Eden, prime minister in the fifties, was a high profile case in point. His CBD was damaged at cholecystectomy. Interestingly, Sir Anthony was transferred to the United States for treatment, which was successful. It led to speculation on the reason for transfer. Surely there were surgeons skilled in this repair in England, or was it just fashionable to think the United States was best? Possibly it was a bit of both in this instance.

On a trip to the United States in 1983, I had visited hospitals in Washington and North Carolina. In the latter, an opportunity arose to examine the operating log of a country-town hospital serving a population of about forty thousand. The log showed that the local general surgeons were only carrying out about three or four operations of any type in a week and only occasionally an operation of the magnitude of an open cholecystectomy. Their experience was therefore very considerably less than that of an English consultant general surgeon. This inexperience meant that injury to the CBD was commoner in the United States than in England, so it follows that tertiary surgeons had more experience in the repair of the resulting problems. Hence the possible reason for Sir Anthony going to the United States for the repair.

Any surgeon skilled in doing Whipple's operation, in which the head or the whole pancreas is excised, is capable of repairing the CBD. In Whipple's operation, the planned division of the CBD and its subsequent anastomosis to the jejunum is part of the operation. I never divided a CBD inadvertently, but did on two occasions carry out reconstructions where others had done so. Both these reconstructions were carried out before the advent of either endoscopic stents for the CBD or laparoscopic surgery. Rubber tubes had to be used as stents, and these caused intense inflammation. A rubber stent can then adhere to the tissue it is in contact with, in this case the CBD. A stent needs to be in place for about three months, to enable healing. The stent keeps the anastomosis open by preventing the scarring process from closing the anastomosis down. Following a Whipple's operation in 1982, the rubber stent that I used at that time did stick to the CBD of one patient and a laparotomy was necessary to free it. Later, inert silastic T-tube stents were available and used in Whipple's operation. After three months in place, they easily slide out and can be removed in the outpatients' department.

f. Biliary surgery,—cholecystectomy, the change from open to laparoscopic operations

The first laparoscopic cholecystectomy was carried out in 1985 in Germany, by Dr E. Muhe. This technique was taken up in the United States by a small number of surgeons, but in 1989, there was a setback, as Reddick and Olson reported. CBD injury following laparoscopic cholecystectomy was five times more likely than after an open cholecystectomy. The US government reacted by announcing that surgeons should do at least fifteen laparoscopic cholecystectomies under supervision before being allowed to do the procedure on their own. This measure reduced the incidence of CBD injury, and laparoscopic cholecystectomy spread worldwide over a very short period in the nineties. It was extraordinary how quickly a new approach for doing an old operation became the standard procedure, and it may even represent the fastest change in technique recorded (table 4).

However, if during a laprascopic cholecystectomy the anatomy of the common bile duct was not clear due to inflammation or adhesions, I converted to an open operation to avoid inadvertently damaging it. This was the safe thing to do. With increasing experience with this technique and constant improvement of the instruments, the conversion rate fell. All patients had to consent to both procedures. The effect of the laparoscopic surgery on bed occupancy was immediate. Initially patients were kept for an overnight stay only. Soon the patients were admitted as day cases compared to the four- or five-day stay in hospital after an open operation, followed by a long convalescence. The benefit of the laparoscopic approach was proved, with postoperative pain reduced to a minimum, as the rate of recovery is dictated by the length of the abdominal wound and is not significantly affected by the extent of the internal operation. It was very unusual, but the laparoscopic approach, was spread by acclaim, as the advantages were so obvious. The instrument designers and manufacturers facilitated this rapid change by significantly ramping up production, so instruments were available when the surgeons needed them, representing another technological advance.

TABLE 4

A. = Open cholecystomies										
B. = Laprascopic cholecystectomies										
	1980	1981	1982	1983	1984	1985	1988	1990	1995	1999	2000
---	---	---	---	---	---	---	---	---	---	---	---
A	37	65	51	81	69	53	98	69	15	2	6
B	0	0	0	0	0	0	0	0	57	30	42

Table 4. Row A shows open cholecystectomies over twenty years. A significant number were carried out annually between 1981 and 1990, dropping to 15 in 1995. The small numbers in 1995, 1999 and 2000 represent conversions from laparoscopic operations while the successfully completed laparoscopic operations are shown in the row below. This illustrates the rapidity of the change in technique. This table is an extract from ch.10 table10.

g. Gut surgery,—the oesophagus

In 1980, there was an ancient rigid brass oesophagoscope in the operating theatres that had not been used for years. It was then put to good use, as I had learned and practised the technique with Mr Bolton-Carter at Leicester. The rigid oesophagoscope was a truly fearsome instrument and could not be used on patients with significant cervical spondylosis, as the cervical spine had to be supple enough to be fully extended to align the mouth and oesophagus. This is also an accomplishment essential for sword swallowers to avoid injuring themselves. The rigid oesophagoscope could only be used with the patient under anaesthetic.

On occasion, an oesophageal cancer was visible using this instrument and it was possible to take a biopsy. If a subsequent chest X-ray showed no obvious sign of spread of the disease, and the biopsy confirmed the diagnosis of cancer, the next test was to do a barium swallow to assess the length of the tumour. If it was less than five centimetres in length then an exploratory laparotomy was arranged, as most tumours less than five centimetres in length could be excised. This was not the same thing as being cured, but it could give some patients reasonable palliation. If the cancer was longer than five centimetres, the tumour was deemed inoperable, as experience had shown this to be so. These were the sum of investigations available in the early eighties.

If at laparotomy a tumour was so advanced that it was adherent to the surrounding tissues, making excision impossible, then a gastrotomy, an opening into the stomach was made. The anaesthetist would pass a tube—designed by Messrs Mousseau and Babin[2] in 1956—through the mouth and slide its long thin tail past the cancer in the oesophagus into the stomach. This would be pulled down by the surgeon, until the wider part of the tube was pulled through the tumour and into the stomach. In this way, the upper end, with a wide funnel top, came to lie just above the carcinoma, and the lower end of the tube proper was then cut to a suitable length so it opened into the stomach. This tube prevented the tumour from obstructing the oesophagus and enabled the patient to eat, albeit a liquidised diet. One patient in whom I had inserted a Mousseau-Babin tube disappeared from follow-up only to be admitted to hospital eighteen months later, where she died shortly thereafter. She had enjoyed a remission, during which she travelled the world for fifteen of those eighteen months. There was no suitable chemotherapy for such tumours at that time, so this was a remarkable result for simple palliation.

However, if at laparotomy the oesophageal cancer was operable, then the stomach was first dissected free, to prepare it to be drawn up into the chest later in the operation to bridge the gap caused by the excision of the cancer. The abdominal wound was then closed. After turning the patient onto the left-hand side, the right side of the chest was opened, and the cancer was freed and excised. The stomach, which had been freed earlier, was then gently pulled into the chest and sutured to the open lower end of the divided oesophagus. In the early eighties, the anastomosis was hand-sewn using wire, but by the mideighties, all these anastomoses were accomplished with stapling devices that were relatively easy to use and gave good results. In most of the patients I operated upon, the presentation was very late, and in most of them the tumour had already spread beyond the confines of the oesophagus. Therefore, this was usually palliative surgery or insertion of a Mousseau-Babin tube. In the eleven years for which I have complete records, twenty-four Mousseau-Babin[2] tubes were inserted. (ch. 10 table 10).

By the mid to late eighties, therapeutic endoscopy was developing rapidly, as mentioned earlier, and cancer of the oesophagus was now diagnosed using a flexible endoscope. The endoscope then was used to assess the mobility of the tumour and to take a biopsy to confirm the diagnosis. A CT scanner was installed at Wigan in 1989 following extensive fund-raising, in which my wife, Sara, took an active part, and then an MRI scan came on line in the early nineties. It was now possible to stage a tumour with much greater accuracy and plan what was to be done in advance of surgery. This was also more humane for the patients, as they would know before surgery what was to be done and were then able to make an informed decision before consenting to the operation.

If these investigations showed the tumour was inoperable, then by use of a special endoscope, a tube much wider than the lumen of the Mousseau-Babin tube could be used to stent the cancer and be left in place. The patient could now swallow in the same way as with the Mousseau-Babin tube, but without having the physiological trauma of an operation that would not improve the prognosis. Another advantage was the relative shortness of the endoscopically placed stent, improving ease of swallowing. It also got blocked less frequently. Once the wide stent was in place, then other forms of treatment, such as radiotherapy and chemotherapy, could be considered, as advances in these treatments began to improve outcomes. Most important, all patients who had undergone only a palliative resection of their oesophagus needed a full three months to recover from the operation, a length of time they could ill afford, considering the very poor prognosis. It was good to abandon the Mousseau-Babin tube once its usefulness was superseded.

h. Gut surgery,—screening for colonic cancer

Within weeks of taking up the appointment of consultant surgeon, it became obvious that in the hospital catchment area, patients with cancer of the colon or rectum almost always presented late in the course of the disease. This was quantified in a collaborative study by twelve surgeons in the North West between May 1981 and July 1983. Five hundred cases of cancer of the colon were analysed. Fifty had been operated on by me. Data was collected to answer two questions. First, how advanced were the colonic cancers when operated on, and second, if the tumours were advanced at operation, why the long delay in coming to surgery?

The result of the survey was revealing and confirmed the observation that in the Wigan Health Authority only 6% of patients coming to operation were classified as Dukes' Stage A, (table 5), while for the North West group as a whole, Dukes' A, was 9%, and in some districts in the South East of England it was as high as 18%. It was alarming to find that Wigan had the lowest number of cancers presenting at the earliest stage of the disease in the North West and probably in the whole country. It can be seen in table 5 that exactly half my patients were staged as Dukes' B, which only carried a 60% five-year survival. Worse, 22% were Dukes' C, with less than a 20% five-year survival rate, and last, 11% were Dukes' D, signifying metastasised cancer, so none were expected to survive five years. With surgery as the only form of treatment available in the eighties, this survival rate in Wigan could only improve the earlier the diagnosis was made and the surgery done.

TABLE 5

Table 5 (i)	Number	Mean age	Age range
Men	29	65	43-84
Women	21	66	41-82

Table 5 (ii).					
Stage of bowel cancer (Dukes)	A	B	C	D	Not Known
50 patients. 1981-1983.	3=6%	25=50%	10=20%	11=22%	1 = 2%
Expected five year survival	97%	60%	22%	0%	-

Table 5. (i) North West of England's Large Bowel Cancer Study 1981–1983: Study of 50 consecutive cases operated on by the author: **(ii)** Stage of cancer at operation with expected cure rates. Only 6 %

had stage A tumours with the best prognosis. Tumours were located as follows: appendix 1, colon 22, rectum 26, anus 1.

Investigation revealed that the majority of patients delayed going to their GP until they had developed symptoms of rectal bleeding and/or a change of bowel habit and abdominal pain. Many had these obvious symptoms for between three and nine months and 20% had delayed approaching their GP for up to a year. This contrasted with the average time lapse from consulting their GP until the actual date of operation, which was only thirty days. The thirty days included outpatient consultation, including rigid sigmoidoscopy, biopsy if appropriate on the first consultation, and investigations including X-rays. This routine ensured that all cancers of the rectum were diagnosed at this first consultation. These patients were given a date for operation at this first attendance, which would be within a fortnight at most. The X-rays of those patients who had diagnostic barium enemas were sent to my secretary's office as soon as completed, where I reviewed them. If a cancer was identified, the patient would be given an appointment at my next outpatients, and when seen all arrangements for the operation were made.

If a GP rang with a patient suspected of having cancer or who was ill, they would be seen the same day if I had a clinic, or in my next clinic if the patient's condition could reasonably wait. If the general practitioner said that the patient's clinical condition was such that they should be seen as a matter of urgency, I would carry out a domiciliary visit in the evening. In patients suspected of having a rectal cancer a sigmoidoscopy and biopsy was carried out during the domiciliary visit, as disposable rigid sigmoidoscopes were available in the early eighties. If the problem was more urgent, with the cancer beginning to obstruct or already obstructing the bowel, then they would be admitted directly to the infirmary.

Three out of the fifty of my colorectal cancer group took much longer to come to surgery after referral by their GP. This was due to difficulty in making the diagnosis in two patients, both ultimately found to have carcinomas of the caecum. The difficulty here was to adequately visualise the caecum by means of a barium enema, after contrast failed to reach the caecum on the first attempt, the barium enema needed to be repeated with inevitable delays. It was not clear why there were delays in making the diagnosis in the third case. Colonoscopy was not available at that time.

TABLE 6

A = Colorectal cancers										
B = Ulcerative colitis including pan-procto colectomy										
C = Ileo-anal pouch formation. Parks Operation										
D = Resections for Crohns disease.										
	1980	1981	1982	1983	1984	1985	1988	1990	1995	1999	2000
A	34	28	29	36	34	40	39	49	16	30	31
B	1	2	1	7	4	8	6	7	10	4	11
C	0	0	0	1	0	0	0	0	0	5	1
D	4	1	3	2	5	2	6	8	2	7	13

Table 6 *shows the numbers of patients undergoing major surgery carried out for bowel cancer and inflammatory bowel disease. This is an extracted from ch. 10 table 10.*

The survey result (table 5), showing very late presentation of patients with bowel cancer, demanded further action. I informed the GPs by post of these findings and also spoke to many individually and also gave a lecture in the Wigan Medical Institute. The lecture was attended by sixty or seventy GPs, who were asked to encourage their patients to seek advice early if they had symptoms. Several of the general practices issued leaflets to their patients. This exercise was repeated regularly over the next few years, with no increase in the numbers of patients with early cancer presenting. Meanwhile, the prepublication results of a trial screening for cancer of the colon in the United States looked very promising and pointed to a way forward.

This trial[3] was published in 1993 and studied 46,000 patients, who either had a test for occult blood in their faeces, using the haemoccult (FOB) test or were randomised to a control group. Controls would not have the FOB test, but would be seen every other year in a clinic. If symptomatic, they would be examined and investigated for cancer, which if diagnosed would be treated in the normal way. This protocol was followed for thirteen years. Those patients with positive FOBs were invited to undergo colonoscopy, by which the diagnosis of cancer, if present, was confirmed and a biopsy taken. The trial, using the FOB test, was successful in identifying many cancers earlier than in the control group. By using this simple screening test, the mortality from cancer in the FOB tested group was reduced by 33% compared to the control group. This was an impressive reduction in mortality, especially as the screening test was simple to use and cost was a trifle, when compared to the cost of screening for other cancers.

With the American trial results available, it seemed logical to start screening for colorectal cancer in Wigan as soon as possible to reduce the dismal late presentation and high mortality from the disease in our area. The general practitioners in two of the largest practices in Wigan with 35,000 patients between them were very enthusiastic to start screening using the FOB test. Our planned protocol in the first year was to target all men who reached their sixtieth birthday in 1996. It was calculated there would be 250 men in this group. Screening, in subsequent years, would be offered to more patients, gradually rolling out the programme to all of the high risk groups. Any patient with a positive FOB would be retested after abstaining from meat for a week. If the test was still positive, they would be offered a colonoscopy in our gastro-enterology department.

The GPs ordered the haemoccult test packs but then hit a bureaucratic brick wall. Alas, the regional health authority refused permission for the GPs to spend the money on the haemoccult tests. The reason given was that there was a trial in progress in England to test the efficacy of the haemoccult test, and until the results were known, permission for such an expense could not be permitted. It was rumoured that the government of the day found it considerably cheaper to give a university department a large sum of money to repeat the American work rather than spend the much larger sum of money on setting up the screening process nationally. To be fair to the university, the research did give the opportunity to work out how to handle a large screening programme that could then be rolled out nationally, but even so it caused an unnecessary delay in starting screening in an area with such a late presentation of the disease.

The results of the English or Nottingham trial published in 1996[4] were impressive with 152,000 patients divided into an FOB-tested group and a control group. Screening for cancer in this trial gave a qualified reduction in mortality of 18% in the tested group. Also in 1996, a Danish group led by O. Kronborg[5] published a trial similar to the American one involving more than 60,000 patients, again divided into FOB-tested patients and controls. This also resulted in a reduction of mortality of 18% in the tested group.

The screening of patients in Wigan finally started in 2007, 11 years after the earlier proposed screening programme was aborted and six years after I had retired. Colonic cancer, of all the common cancers, is the easiest and cheapest to identify by screening due to the long latent period between the development of a colonic polyp and its progression to malignancy. Removal of polyps prevents development of a cancer, and resection of an early cancer has a cure rate of 95% or higher. Successful screening will also lead to less complex surgery. There have also been significant advances in preoperative radiotherapy, especially for cancer of the rectum, in recent years. Table 6 shows my firm's work-load for major gut surgery.

Due to the late presentation of the disease (table 6) many of the colonic resections carried out were complex operations, the tumour having infiltrated the surrounding tissues. These operations were lengthy, compared to a resection of a Dukes A tumour, and could involve excision of other organs which had been infiltrated. Also, for example, if the ureter needed stenting to prevent damaging it because it was embedded in tumour tissue, I could accomplish this without delay.

i. Gut Surgery,—gastric surgery and surgery for duodenal ulcers

Carcinoma of the stomach was common, as can be seen in table 7. The commonest operation was a partial gastrectomy, as first described and carried out by Billroth in 1881. If the cancer involved the whole stomach, then a total gastrectomy was carried out and the gap between the lower oesophagus and duodenum was bridged with a pouch formed from small bowel (ilium), using the technique I had learned from Mr Slack at the Middlesex Hospital. This was a great advance on simply interposing a section of small bowel, as the pouch was a reservoir. Patients could return to eating normally, as those cured by the operation demonstrated.

The rationale and progress in treatment for duodenal ulcer is described in chapter 6. The cure is now achieved by eradication of Helicobacter pylori infection by medical means, making surgery obsolete. This is clearly shown in table 7, where these operations are in decline from 1988. The last vagotomy I performed was in 1990. This sophisticated operation cured most sufferers but left a small number of patients with significant side effects such as dumping syndrome. That, in turn, required revision surgery, which can also be seen in table 7; the last such operation was also carried out in 1990.

TABLE 7

A = Gastrectomy for cancer
B = Vagotomy and Pyloroplasty (V&P)
C = Revision gastrectomy for complications of V&P.

	1980	1981	1982	1983	1984	1985	1988	1990	1995	1999	2000
A	9	21	19	16	21	8	20	17	4	7	10
B	12	8	11	18	12	10	5	1	0	0	0
C	4	2	4	8	5	3	0	2	0	0	0

Table 7 shows that cancer of the stomach was quite common and provided a steady work-load. Vagotomy and pyloroplasty for duodenal ulcer disease began to taper off in 1988 following the identification of Helicobacter pylori as a cause of duodenal ulcer and its susceptibility to antibiotics. There were no V&Ps after 1990. The revision gastrectomies after V&P were all, except one problems the author inherited and included 4 with recurrent ulcer, 3 with dumping syndrome and the rest with pyloric stenosis. This is an extract from ch. 10 table10.

j. Audit of inguinal hernia repair

In the early nineties, inguinal hernia repairs were audited at Wigan. The result was not unexpected but salutary. In my firm about 15% of all inguinal hernia repairs each year were for recurrent hernias, a few recently done but most old repairs. Maloney's darn had been the standard method of repair, and the results were poor when compared with the Shouldice repair, mentioned in an earlier chapter.

Mr Tony Blower and I arranged to receive training to carry out inguinal hernia repairs laparoscopically, using the intraperitoneal approach to try to improve the success of hernia repair. After excising the hernial sac, a mesh was fixed over the defect left by the hernia. The continuity of the peritoneum was then restored, covering the mesh and separating it from the abdominal cavity. The results were uniformly good. Neither of us had any complications, but we recognised that in these very early days of laparoscopic hernia repair, any complication from this approach would be major—causing damage to a major blood vessel, for instance. We judged that it was better to continue with the inguinal approach until such time as new instrumentation and information made this approach more acceptable.

These problems were illustrated by two patients referred to me for laparoscopic hernia repair. The first was a middle-aged man with chronic renal failure. I explained to him that, although the risk of complications was low, any complication would be serious and could have an impact on his renal failure, which might then be life-threatening. He could not accept this, as he wanted to be back at work the day after surgery. I offered a minimal inguinal approach under local anaesthetic; he declined and went elsewhere. The second was a twenty-year-old woman, about to be married, looking forward to having a family. I explained that an unnecessary intra-abdominal repair was unwise and offered a repair as above. She accepted and the result was excellent.

A while later Mr Tony Blower, Mr Hakim Azmi, who had formerly been my registrar and was at that time an associate specialist and later a consultant general surgeon at Wigan, and I travelled to the London Hernia Centre to observe a mesh repair using an inguinal incision, which had been pioneered in the United States by Lichtenstein. We were impressed, and at the following routine surgical audit at the RAEI we persuaded our colleagues that all inguinal hernias in Wigan should be carried out using this method. This agreement was quite a triumph and the first time a unified policy for treatment for any condition was achieved as, in the past, one of my colleagues had always refused to be bound by such agreements.

Hakim Azmi offered to teach and supervise all new registrars and SHOs in the Lichtenstein technique and set to work. The initial results a year later showed no recurrence to date. Later audit showed that the rate of recurrence had dropped to 1%, a pleasing improvement for the patients and Hakim Azmi, who had worked diligently to ensure that Lichtenstein's technique was applied as described.

k. Training surgical registrars

The model used for training my registrars was that learned from Mr John Marsh in Warwick (table 1) and Professor Peter Bell in Leicester. This was in practice a true apprenticeship. All registrars who came to work for me were fellows of the Royal College of Surgeons (FRCS), and all had practical experience. In the eighties, several were promoted to registrar after working as senior house officer in Wigan or Leigh.

My first two registrars, Mr Paul Chui in Wigan and Mr Bhatnager in Leigh, were very experienced and capable of operating safely to a high level, including such operations as straightforward colectomies and gastrectomies. Both benefitted from the introduction of vascular and oesophageal surgery to the district.

I then appointed Mr Tomy Shafy as my registrar at Wigan, a very capable young surgeon who had qualified in Egypt. As my former SHO, he set to work in his new post with a will. To begin with, he assisted at operations. Then I assisted him on selected tasks during operations. As confidence in his capabilities increased, he operated on selected cases with me present in the theatre complex. Quite frequently I would go into his theatre to look over his shoulder to see how things were going and of course assist if the going was difficult. He always asked for advice immediately on meeting a situation beyond his experience. This was vital, especially at night, for emergencies who had been admitted through A&E, or for any of my in-patients who were causing concern, whether or not I was officially on duty.

If rung concerning one of my patients, by knowing what operation had been carried out I would have a very clear idea of what the problem was. I could decide what action should be taken, either by the registrar or by my going into the hospital. This is the essence of continuity of care. Patients are known, and time does not need to be wasted in an urgent situation by going through the preliminaries as with a new patient. The problem then receives immediate attention and any further operation if needed is done as a matter of urgency.

This pattern of training was followed for all subsequent registrars until the late nineties. For many years, a new registrar's first six months of an appointment resulted in frequent calls for my advice or help. The frequency of these calls then naturally decreased, and by the time the registrar had been in post for nine months, he or she had become a very useful surgeon. Not only were they learning and gaining experience but also providing an excellent service to the NHS. For example, as a registrar progressed, he or she was given one operating list a week over several months dedicated to intermediate operations. This built confidence in the handling of tissues and the registrar learned that not all such operations are straightforward, while help from his or her chief was always at hand.

There were still twin operating lists under my control. This arrangement was not only approved of, but it was considered to be the best of tools for training registrars. In 1998, the use of twin operating theatres to teach and give experience to registrars fell out of favour with some senior medical people in the Royal Colleges and NHS management. The latter, directed by government, were accelerating the taking over of day-to-day control of the NHS, and all dual lists were abolished. This, and the reduction of operating lists available to me from six a week to three, had a dramatic effect on the volume of work that the firm could undertake. This is seen in ch 10, table 10, where the average of elective operations between 1980 and 1995 was 878 per annum and then fell to 332 per annum, a reduction of 62%.

Table 8

Classification of operations by complexity (BUPA) and weighting for comparisons of work-load	
CMO = Complex Major Operations	4 POINTS
M+ = Major Plus operations	2.2 POINTS
M = Major operations	1.75 POINTS
I = Intermediate operations	1 POINT
Minor operations	0.5 POINT

124

Table 8. *The British United Provident Association's (BUPA) 1990 classification of operations was used by the Royal College of Surgeons to make comparisons of work-load for each of five categories of operation of decreasing complexity. Each category is given a different numerical weighting. This classification is used in table 9.*

In the early eighties, this retrograde change was still years away. So these first nine months involved intensive training. By the end of this period, all my registrars were able to operate solo on selected cases with confidence, both mine and theirs, which meant that my registrar had "come of age." At this point I was able to manage my three operating lists every Thursday in the same way that Professor Peter Bell had used his theatres in Leicester.

For example, in 1992 my registrars were Mr T. P. N. Udaya-Kumar, who moved on in the middle of the year and was succeeded by Mr I. Boughdady. Between them they operated on 464 patients, representing 38% of the total elective operating load of the firm (see table 9). The breakdown of these operations by complexity was that 9 of them were CMOs, 22 major+ and 99 major operations, and the rest were intermediate and minor procedures (see table 8). My SHO at the start of that year was Dr S. Balaji, who carried out 203 operations representing just less than 17% of the total. Then Dr Florence Geers took over later in the year and operated on 57 patients (4.6%). So the SHOs carried out a great deal of work and were responsible for just over 21%, or 256 operations. Of these, 28 were major, and 79 were intermediate operations. This pattern and wealth of experience gained by the registrars and SHOs took place between 1981 and 1998.

Every month, all the consultant surgeons with their firms met for an audit meeting. These meetings were greatly aided in the midnineties by an extremely able and helpful statistician. Every few months, he produced a graph of "who had done what" in my firm for the previous month. This covered analysis of morbidity, mortality, and complications. Training was also reviewed.

The statistics showed the progress made in 1995 by my registrar Mr Vince Smyth. He proved to be a very able surgeon and took full advantage of the opportunities with which he was presented. In February, he was responsible for only 13 of the 108 elective operations carried out by the firm, representing 8.66% of the total. In December he topped the list, operating on 38 of the 92 patients, including 7 in the major+ category, in all representing 40.11% of the firm's operative work-load, with an intermediate equivalent score (IEQ) of 44.9 (see table 8). This showed good progress as a surgeon when compared to the February total but also the accumulation of considerable and broad-based experience in both elective and emergency surgery.

TABLE 9

Operating workload of Author's Firm for the whole year of 1992.						
Operation by Organ			BUPA category			
	CMO	Major+	Major	Inter	Minor	Totals
Colon	19	32	29	47	155	282
Skin	0	0	1	22	139	162
Abdominal	1	16	118	12	3	150
Hernia	2	0	12	128	0	142
Genito-urinary	0	0	3	48	32	83
Varicose Veins.	0	0	0	75	7	82
Stomach	7	13	44	3	0	67
Appendix	0	0	63	2	0	65
Arterial	39	4	11	1	1	56
Thyroid/Parathyroid	0	0	33	5	0	38
Breast	0	0	5	23	1	29
Amputations	0	0	23	1	0	24
Miscellaneous	1	1	9	6	8	25
Lymphatics	0	0	2	11	1	14
TOTALS	69	66	253	384	347	1219

Table 9 shows the total operating load of 1219 operations, both elective and emergency, undertaken by my firm in 1992 which was a typical year. The work-load is broken down into broad categories. Gastro-intestinal operations (colon+abdominal+stomach+appendix) accounted for just over 46% of the total. Vascular surgery, including both arterial and varicose vein surgery, weighed in at just over 13%, typical of a general surgical firm. To see a more detailed breakdown of elective operations only, please look at chapter 10, table 10.

l. Registrar appointments

In 1998, district general hospitals (DGHs) were no longer allowed to appoint their own registrars. All the new registrars at the RAEI were then appointed by the teaching hospitals and rotated out to the DGHs for a fixed appointment of six months. It was then that the first female registrar was appointed to my firm who was excellent. The only reason that I had not appointed a woman sooner was that none had applied.

To place this in perspective, when I was a student, only 15% of my year, both at Oxford and St Thomas's, were women. Now the current intake of women into some medical schools in Britain is over 60%. A majority of women in the profession will be reflected in the future as the sex ratio of doctors changes strongly in favour of women. As they climb the rungs of seniority, women will dominate in the twenty-first century in comparison to the male dominance of the twentieth century and before.

In 2009, the Royal College of Physicians published online an investigation titled, "Women in Medicine, the Future." This concluded that entry to medical school appears to be on a meritocratic basis. "Nevertheless, white males are now under-represented. This is relative to their share of the relevant age group amongst medical school applicants, and to an even greater extent than they are in higher education generally."

Why this might be so is not clear and deserves fuller examination. A snapshot of the situation in 2007, with respect to the number of women in the UK medical profession, shows the following: (i) women made up 57% of both applicants and acceptances for medical schools, and (ii) women made up approximately 40% of all qualified doctors, this subdivided as 42% of all GPs and 28% of all consultants in the NHS in England.

m. Training of registrars and the European Working Time Directive, EWTD 1998

The European Working Time Directive[6] came into force in October 1998. It became compulsory for junior doctors in 2003 but was implemented in many hospitals by 1999. There were some exceptions, but this did not include trainee doctors, where the regulation clearly lays down, "If you are a trainee doctor, the forty-eight-hour maximum working hours applies to you." For the NHS to comply in reducing the hours worked by junior doctors to an average of forty-eight hours a week over seventeen weeks it was necessary for them to work a shift system, in order that patient cover in hospitals could be maintained twenty-four hours a day all year round. The EU directive de facto put an end to the old system of hospital doctors working in firms. With the demise of the firm went continuity of care and the apprenticeship, which had served surgeons well for nearly one hundred and thirty years.

The typical registrar's cycle of rotation in 1999 started with night duty, usually twelve-hour shifts for seven days. One might have anticipated that this would lead to the gaining of much valuable experience with admitting emergencies and operating. However, by 2000 very little operating was carried out at night, except for life-threatening emergencies such as severe haemorrhage. Such emergencies as ectopic pregnancy or even leaking aortic aneurysms are not that common, so they provide little experience for the registrar.

Cases of peritonitis, incarcerated or strangulated hernias, or appendicitis, to mention a few common examples, would be admitted, rehydrated, and treated with antibiotics overnight. Such patients were listed for operation the next morning on an emergency/trauma list staffed by a consultant surgeon and a consultant anaesthetist. The registrar who had looked after these patients overnight would greatly benefit from being present at, assisting at, or operating during the morning list for experience, and also to see if his or her diagnoses were correct. This did not occur, because the registrars had to leave the hospital and go home at the end of their shift.

The second week of the rota was a break at home after working long shifts for a week. Thus the second week did not add to professional development.

The third week consisted of working nine to five from Monday to Friday. Then, if what occurred in the RAEI after I retired was commonplace, the consultants had two half-day lists each week in which to practise and teach surgery. Registrars are struggling to gain adequate experience. In addition, they do not have the opportunity to benefit from, or gain satisfaction by doing service work.

The hours worked by the registrar in the three-week rota described above total 128 hours on duty, of which only eight hours are in the operating theatre. Then there is evidence presented by Lord Darzi[7] that training has been reduced from 80,000 to 6,000 hours.

In practice, it has proved challenging to adequately train the next generation of surgeons, as was frequently expressed by Mr John Black[8], president of the Royal College of Surgeons (2008–2011). He wrote how continuity of care was completely absent, and a patient could be seen by: consultant A on first attending outpatients; consultant B on follow-up with tests and scans; if an operation is indicated, consultant C would operate; and if the patients were lucky enough to have a follow up appointment, then he or she would be seen by consultant D.

John Black worked tirelessly as president of the Royal College of Surgeons to persuade government to obtain derogation from the European Working Time Directive for surgeons-in-training. Such derogation would enable the training of the current generation of registrars to be improved by increased experience. In spite of his tremendous effort this has not been successful to date.

n. The grand round and its demise

Another casualty of the changes was the grand round. Between 1980 and 1998 my firm's grand round was always on a Wednesday afternoon. During that morning, students clerked all the patients admitted for the operating lists on the Thursday, when there was one all-day list and a second morning list in tandem. For many years, there were up to forty inpatients under my care on Wednesdays, being a mix of those admitted as emergencies, postoperative patients, and those for surgery the following day. All were presented to the grand round. The whole afternoon was thus spent talking to and examining each patient, and discussing signs, symptoms, operations, and postoperative care of each one. In fact, every aspect of the management of the surgical patient was discussed.

By the end of the afternoon, the whole firm were familiar with all the patients, and as we moved from bed to bed, the opportunity to mark the side or site of an operation with an indelible marker was taken. This was always done in discussion with the patient, so there were never any mistakes with operations being performed on the wrong side or site. The experience that everyone gained was wide, encompassing endocrine, vascular, hepato-biliary, pancreatic, upper gastro-intestinal, colorectal, and paediatric surgery, both elective and emergency. The registrars especially gained as their opinions were sought, and they would also tell the round of new techniques and procedures they had learned from meetings and grand rounds at the teaching hospitals. In turn, I learned a lot from the registrars. Wednesday afternoons were the highlight of the week.

The grand round finally ceased in early 1998 due to lack of beds to admit patients the day before their operation. This was seen as a luxury by management, who did not take into account the value to the care of patients and teaching.

Another problem caused by only admitting a patient to the ward on the morning of the operation is that there may or may not be a bed available. This means the patient might sit in the ward's day-room, hoping that a bed becomes available, for if not, the hapless patient is discharged home to go through the whole process again.

It was also noticeable that, between 1980 and 1989, the number of geriatric patients admitted both for elective and emergency procedures increased by about 2% a year; this, coupled with the halving of the beds available in hospital, resulted in the occupation of beds exceeding 100% at times. Geriatric was defined as the patients over sixty-five. I know that this pressure on beds has increased considerably since and will continue to do so in the twenty-first century.

o. **Finances**

The cost of the NHS doubled after 2000 from sixty billion pounds annually to over one hundred and fifty billion in 2008.[9] Consultants received a pay rise in 2003–4. This resulted in a consultant in his or her first year of appointment receiving a salary of £74,500. I was replaced by three consultants, so the work that used to be done by my firm is now costing nearly four hundred percent more in salaries—all within a few years of my retirement. Overall, the increase in the number of consultant surgeons at the trust has more than doubled.

The sense of ownership of patients is very important. I can remember as a registrar feeling that the patients were mine as well as my chief's. In years gone by, the senior doctors would have shut wards, as I did on one occasion in Wigan in the early eighties, when nursing levels were not safe. In the target culture of the NHS, this is not possible. The consultants now appear to have little control over the spending of money. The deterioration started in the seventies when the then-secretary of state for health, Lady Barbara Castle, removed control of budgets from the consultant hospital management committees. It took another twenty-five years for management to wrest the last vestiges of control of the finances from the medical profession.

p. References

1. Lee, H. H. Bacterial Charity Work leads to population wide resistance. *Nature* 467 (Sept. 2010): 82–85.
2. Mousseau, M., J. Forestier, J. Babin, and M. Hardy. Place de l'intubation a demeure dans le traitment palliatif du cancer de l'oesophage. *Archives Mal. Appar. Dig Mal Nutr.* 45 (1956): 208-214.
3. Mandel, J., J. Bond, T. Church, et al. "Reducing Mortality from Colorectal Cancer by Screening for Faecal Occult Blood: Minnesota Colon Cancer Control Study." *New Eng. J. of Med.* 328 (1993): 1365–1371.
4. Hardcastle, J., J. Chamberlain, M. Robinson, et al. "Randomised Controlled Trial of Faecal-Occult-Blood Screening for Colorectal Cancer." *Lancet* 348 (1996): 1472–1477.

5. Kronborg, O., C. Fenger, J. Olsen, et al. "Randomised Study of Screening for Colorectal Cancer with Faecal-Occult-Blood Test." *Lancet* 348 (1996): 1467–1471.

6. EU Working Time Directive 2003/88/EC. In the NHS doctors had been required to work unfeasibly long hours on call. (I am sure unreasonably long hours was meant, they were always feasible if unsociable! Author).

7. Bann, S., and A. Darzi. "Selection of Individuals for Training in Surgery." *Am. J. Surg* 190 (2005): 98–102.

8. Black, J., President's Newsletter: The College at the Party conferences. Ann Roy *Coll Surg Eng (suppl)* 2009; 91: 294–295. .

9. NHS funding and expenditure 1950–2010/11. H&C Library SN/SG/724 Updated 03/04/ General Statistics Table 4.

CHAPTER 10

Table 10: Author's Operations 1980-2000

	1980	1981	1982	1983	1984	1985	1988	1990	1995	1999	2000
Amputations of limbs	2	5	3	7	7	5	12	19	18	11	5
Aneurysm aortic	3	8	4	5	3	5	10	13	11	12	7
Fem pop/axillo-femoral bypass	4	6	6	3	12	13	7	9	16	9	0
Aortfem bypass uni/bilateral	2	3	15	13	15	16	14	12	20	0	3
False aneurysm repair	0	0	0	0	0	0	0	0	1	2	1
ExcCervRib/Sympathectomy	1	0	1	0	2	1	1	0	2	0	0
Breast Local excision	26	8	33	53	42	30	12	9	3	0	0
Mastectomy	18	21	9	21	9	8	6	0	6	0	0
Breast biopsy	14	30	7	5	16	11	26	3	1	0	0
Microdochectomy	3	7	4	3	2	5	2	2	1	0	0
Gynecomastia	0	0	3	0	2	1	0	1	0	0	0
Colo-rectal carcinoma	34	28	29	36	34	40	39	49	16	30	31
Ulcerativecolitis, colectomy/pan-proctocolectomy	1	2	1	7	4	8	6	7	10	4	11
Endometriosis	1	0	0	0	0	0	0	0	0	0	0
Polyposis coli	0	0	0	0	0	0	0	1	0	0	0
Actinomycosis, colonic resection	1	0	0	0	0	0	0	0	0	0	0
sarcoma/melanoma excision	1	0	0	0	0	0	0	2	0	1	0
Ilio-anal pouch formation	0	0	0	1	0	0	1	5	0	2	1
Crohns diseaseresections	4	1	3	2	5	2	6	8	2	7	13
Colectomy for megacolon	0	0	0	0	1	0	0	0	0	2	0
Diverticular disease colectomy	2	1	2	2	1	1	1	0	0	5	1
Colo/recto-vesical fistula operations	0	6	3	2	2	4	0	1	1	1	0

Rectal prolapse operations	2	2	2	9	1	0	0	0	0	2	2
Hartmann's operation reversal	0	0	1	0	1	1	0	2	0	1	2
Appendicectomy/interval	6	0	3	6	7	5	4	0	1	4	5
Colostomy/ileostomy formationand revision	6	10	12	9	18	12	10	15	8	3	4
York Mason's/transanal op	2	1	0	0	0	0	0	1	0	0	0
Haemorrhoids	7	1	5	10	17	11	21	20	11	9	8
Resection following irradiation of small bowel	0	0	3	2	0	0	0	1	0	0	0
Fistula-in-ano including Crohns fistulae	0	0	2	17	13	4	0	8	5	13	7
Minor operations	124	74	33	102	130	113	142	176	161	21	12
Minor ano/rectal ops	64	65	60	118	111	139	194	123	54	19	21
Laparoscopy exploratory	0	0	0	0	0	0	0	0	1	0	4
Laparotomy exploratory	12	25	13	24	16	18	40	16	15	9	7
Cholecystectomy open	37	65	51	81	69	53	98	69	15	2	6
Cholecystectomy laparoscopic	0	0	0	0	0	0	0	0	57	30	42
Gallstone ileus	0	0	0	0	0	0	0	0	0	2	0
Common bileduct exploration	0	9	0	12	5	7	15	2	7	0	0
Jaundice laparotomy	11	4	6	8	6	5	3	1	0	0	0
Oesophagoscopy rigid	6	7	0	0	0	0	0	0	0	0	0
Oesophago-gastrectomy	0	0	2	1	9	3	4	5	7	0	0
Gastric carcinoma partial/total gastrectomy	9	21	19	16	21	8	20	17	4	7	10
Revision gastrectomy post V & P	4	2	4	8	5	3	0	2	0	0	0
Gastric ulcer gastrectomy	2	0	2	0	0	0	0	2	0	0	0
Vagotomy & pyloroplasty (V&P)	12	8	11	18	12	10	5	1	0	0	0
Anti reflux operations/HH repair	0	2	4	10	7	4	12	9	6	9	4
Gastric volvulus	0	1	1	0	1	0	0	0	0	0	0
Pyloric stenosis (Ramstedt's op.)	1	1	4	1	2	3	0	0	0	0	0
gastro-jejunostomy	0	0	1	2	0	1	0	0	3	0	2
Moussin-Babin tube insertion	4	1	0	1	1	5	5	6	0	1	0
Feeding gastrostomy	0	0	0	0	0	0	0	2	1	1	1
Circumcision	31	45	26	53	32	26	54	18	26	2	1
Epididymal cyst	1	0	2	2	4	2	4	2	2	0	0
Orchidopexy	20	20	16	19	18	13	25	6	1	0	0
Orchidectomy	1	3	1	4	1	0	6	3	1	0	0

Hydrocele/varicocele	5	6	6	5	3	14	23	12	5	2	1
Cystoscopy	30	11	8	12	6	9	2	0	1	0	0
Urethral dilatation	3	2	1	0	0	0	0	0	0	0	0
Vasectomy/reversal of vasectomy	2	6	0	4	17	19	35	5	17	0	0
Exploration of testis	0	0	2	0	0	0	0	0	0	0	0
Hysterectomy/oophorectomy	0	0	1	1	0	0	0	0	0		0
Nephrectomy	1	0	0	0	0	0	0	0	0		0
Hernia repair (all)	91	104	103	138	132	144	141	147	129	61	57
Melanoma excision	3	1	0	2	2	1	13	0	2	1	2
Rhabdomyosarcoma excision	0	0	0	0	0	0	0	0	1	1	0
Splenectomy elective	1	0	4	0	5	1	0	1	1	5	3
Thyroidectomy carcinoma/nodular	11	14	25	19	27	34	18	23	36	15	21
Parathyroidectomy	2	6	3	3	1	2	2	2	4	8	6
Thyroidectomy hyperthyroidism	0	21	0	0	0	0	0	3	0	6	3
Tracheostomy elective	0	0	0	0	0	0	0	0	0	0	2
Tongue tie division	3	1	1	5	2	5	1	6	7	3	2
Adrenalectomy	0	2	0	1	0	0	0	0	1	0	0
Pancreatic carcinoma (Whipple's operation)	0	1	2	0	1	1	1	4	1	1	0
Pancreatic pseudocyst bypass	2	0	3	1	4	0	0	4	0	0	4
Pilonidal sinus operations	10	10	4	12	13	8	10	9	6	8	10
Branchial cyst, thyroglossal cyst & pharyngeal pouch operations	0	1	3	4	7	4	4	2	4	0	0
Mandibular duct stone	7	1	0	0	2	4	3	2	0	0	0
Varicose vein surgery	64	22	16	50	122	99	68	23	119	10	0
Portocaval shunt	0	1	0	0	0		0	0	0	0	0
TOTALS	714	703	618	986	1042	980	1126	891	843	342	322

Table 10: Presents the operating data for elective surgery for 11 years between 1980 and 2000, when the author was a consultant general and vascular surgeon in Wigan. The years not shown in the table represent an arbitrary exclusion to reduce the volume of records I could take into my retirement. The missing years were not significantly different from the years recorded here. The table shows interesting changes in the practice of surgery due to advances in imaging and instrumentation. The last years, 1999 and 2000, show a significant change, not only in the volume but also the pattern of work, as management changes made a serious impact. The number of operating lists I had at Wigan was reduced from six to three to accommodate new surgeons in subspecialities. All surgery for day cases went to Leigh Infirmary. The traces of these changes can be seen in this table. The appointment of the first surgeon trained in a single area of expertise was a breast surgeon, and the reduction of breast surgery done by my firm can be seen from 1990 onwards. The arrival of a vascular specialist in 1999 is reflected, from that year, in the reduction of my carrying out bypass grafts for arterial obstructive disease.

CHAPTER 11

Private Practice and Independent British Healthcare plc.

In the early eighties, it was considered that all consultants should practice in the same hospital for both their NHS and private practice and would therefore be "geographically whole time." This was a good concept, as consultants would then be on hand throughout the working day for the care of all of their patients.

Adjacent to the Royal Albert Edward Infirmary in Wigan was a small private hospital within a few yards of the main building. Christopher Home had been endowed in the 1930s by Mr Christopher, a generous benefactor. By the time I came to Wigan in 1980, the ground floor of Christopher Home had been taken over by the NHS and converted into the NHS eye unit. However the first floor was still a private ward, with its own operating theatre and 11 private rooms. Christopher Home was cheerfully and efficiently run by a senior sister who was completely dedicated to her work. I was happy to bring private patients there, as and when they might be referred by their GPs. If private operations were needed, then Christopher Home was where they were carried out, and where the patients stayed until they were discharged home. I visited my patients at Christopher Home every morning at seven thirty on my way into the Royal Albert Edward Infirmary fifty yards away and also on my way home. This was an ideal arrangement in early nineteen eighty and there was no reason to think that this arrangement would not continue indefinitely.

This was not to be the case, for within a few months of my arrival in April 1980, the NHS trade unions were threatening strike action. Moreover, as time went by they became increasing bellicose, demanding, amongst other things, that there should be no private beds at all in NHS hospitals. The unions had considerable support from their rank and file, so it was with reluctance that I started to look around to see where else I could admit my private patients.

The choice was either the Alexandra Hospital in Manchester, or Fairfield Hospital in Rainford near St Helens. I opted for the latter. Fairfield Hospital was an attractive modern hospital in the country with excellent facilities, and the care of the patients was good. Unfortunately, there was only one session left in the operating theatre schedule that was free and this clashed with one of my NHS outpatient clinics. This was often inconvenient and meant keeping patients waiting. It caused me some unease, so could only be a temporary arrangement. Another problem was that Fairfield Hospital was relatively remote, being eighteen miles away from home and twenty-two miles from the RAEI. To visit my patients at Fairfield Hospital first thing in the morning meant leaving home at half past six to allow enough time to start my work at the RAEI at eight o'clock. The disadvantages of not being a "geographically whole time consultant" were clear.

My forebodings were correct, and the plan to switch to Fairfield Hospital was judicious, because the unions did call a strike. It proved to be the longest and most disruptive strike that the NHS ever endured, either before or afterwards, and lasted nine whole months.

I had sympathy with the strikers as their pay was poor at that time, but unhappily, their actions put patients at risk in the NHS. The unions forbade the admission of any patient for routine non-urgent operations to the hospital. Patients whose operations were deferred did not disappear, as they still need-ed their operations, and my waiting list built up rapidly. By the end of the strike there were several hundred patients waiting for clinically non-urgent procedures, and all the time referrals continued to pour in.

During the strike, not a single private patient was admitted ei-ther to the infirmary or to Christopher Home. This inconvenience was trivial compared to the effect of the strike on the NHS patients for the reasons given above. With full-time pickets at the gates of the infirmary, the unions set out to enforce their will. Indeed, even patients with conditions needing urgent treatment, although not classified as emergencies, had to have their case argued with the local shop steward.

On one preoperative ward round, I was talking to an elderly pa-tient who had recurrent abdominal pain and needed an urgent di-agnostic investigation to look for and biopsy, if present, a suspected cancer. My registrar, Mr Chui, whispered in my ear "The shop stew-ard asks why this is an emergency, as he does not think you should proceed." After a moment's reflection, I asked Mr Chui to ring the shop steward and ask if he would kindly join us on the ward round. We would all then be able discuss whether to proceed or not with the patient, and if the procedure was to be deferred, then perhaps he would be good enough to explain it to the patient himself. A few min-utes later, I received a message asking me to proceed please. At least the general civilities of life were maintained in these difficult times.

Since the unions had not embargoed operations on children, I took advantage of this to see that all the children on the NHS wait-ing list were operated on quickly, and I encouraged GPs to give me a ring about any child needing an operation. The child would be seen in my next clinic at the RAEI. In this way an operation, if needed, could be arranged within a few days, as at that time consultants had complete control over their waiting lists.

While the strike was underway, my predecessor, Mr William (Bill) Weatherstone-Wilson, who had continued to live locally after retirement, rang me and asked if I would be interested in going to a meeting at Euxton Hall near Chorley. A development company was considering buying it to convert into a convalescent home. He thought that as his successor, I might be interested. I thanked him and said I would go.

The meeting, on Tuesday, 2 February 1982, at 5.30 p.m. was informal, but in reality it was a cocktail party that was hosted by Mrs Margaret Fenton, the owner of Euxton Hall. She had inherited it from her father, Sir Stanley Bell, a cabinet minister in a pre-war Tory government. For generations before this, the hall had been in the possession of the Anderton family, who could boast that one of their ancestors had been the secretary to the Earl of Derby during the Civil War (1642-1651). Later in the nineteenth century, the Andertons gave many valuable documents from that earlier period to the Wigan Town Hall Library. A fire at Euxton Hall in 1929 had severely damaged the house. When it was rebuilt, it was with a single floor only, not counting the huge cellars, and it could best be described as a stately bungalow.

During the Second World War, there was a huge underground munitions factory in the village of Euxton, where thirty-three thousand workers were brought daily by train to work. Lord Haw-Haw, whose real name was William Joyce, was one of several British announcers who broadcasted propaganda from Nazi Germany in a radio programme named *Germany Calling*. In his broadcasts he had frequently mentioned Euxton, threatening its destruction by the Luftwaffe. The locals and workers were always amused by this, as he always mispronounced Euxton as "Yooxton," when every local knows that the U is silent! Joyce was hanged after the war as a traitor.

At the Euxton Hall meeting, the sitting room was packed. A Mr Askew introduced himself to me and talked a lot about nursing home conversions and then asked if I was interested in using a convalescent home for my patients. I said no, but I added that the development of a private hospital would be a different matter. I would certainly use it myself, and I thought that many of my colleagues would also be interested. A few minutes later, Mr Keith Chadwick, a Blackpool businessman who was managing director of Financial and Professional Services Ltd, came over to speak to me. His company was negotiating the purchase of Euxton Hall to convert it into a nursing home. My idea of developing a hospital instead had been relayed to him by Mr Askew and he had thought about it and liked the concept. He could envisage a more promising future for Euxton Hall as a hospital than a nursing home. We had a long discussion, and both of us were enthusiastic about the idea. When we parted he promised to see what could be done; he said that he would be in touch.

During the meeting, my wife Sara was speaking to someone who explained the process needed for planning permission. He was on the local planning committee and surprised Sara by telling her that she could be in a position to help get a planning application passed by the committee. Not being able to think of any way that she would care to help him to get the planning permission passed, she beat a hasty retreat. Interestingly the local authority planning committee did refuse the application, probably on political grounds. Valuable months were lost after the refusal. An appeal made its way to London before planning permission was granted when the matter was voted on by the whole council.

A week after talking to Keith Chadwick, I was surprised to receive an architectural drawing for converting Euxton Hall into a hospital. The plan showed an area of Euxton Hall's courtyard reserved for an operating theatre complex, which was left blank. The speed and professionalism of this response by Mr Chadwick surprised me. It was my first experience of business in the private sector, and this speed was very different from what happened in the NHS. I was also later to discover the power of a board of directors to see a formal decision turned into immediate action, by which I was much impressed.

The drawings for converting Euxton Hall into a hospital were very exciting, and I met Mr Max Elliot the architect. The prospect and timing for developing a private hospital were very good. It would be a place where I could admit private patients for surgery only four miles from my home in Standish and only seven from the Royal Albert Edward Infirmary in Wigan.

After this, Mr Chadwick and his adviser Mr Keith Padgett, formerly with BUPA, met me frequently. Mr Chadwick changed the name of an existing "shell" company to Euxton Hall Independent Hospital Ltd. The company secretary of the "shell" company then resigned, and the first board of directors of Euxton Hall Independent Hospital were appointed. Only two were appointed: Keith Chadwick was the new chairman and I was appointed director. In this way, on 14 June 1982, I became one of the two founding directors of Euxton Hall Independent Hospital Ltd. I then purchased five thousand one-pound shares in the company, the first capital the company received. It is with great pride that I look back to being one of those two founding directors.

Following the inaugural meeting, we met regularly in the evenings at my house in Standish. Keith Chadwick was easy to work with and always met the inevitable difficulties cheerfully and confidently. He had great skill in people management. This latter ability stood the company in good stead when staff recruitment started shortly afterwards.

Sara and I had great fun designing the operating theatre and operating theatre complex for the new hospital. Sara's architectural drawing skills and my knowledge of operating theatres enabled us to provide a detailed design within the space constraints that the courtyard imposed. Until the day that the hospital opened, there was no way of knowing how well the theatre complex would function. In the event, it was the best theatre I ever used, and it continued in daily use unaltered for nearly twenty years, at which time a second theatre was built into the complex.

During the development phase of the hospital, there were discussions with many colleagues from all the different specialities.

Detailed instrument lists were drawn up, and all machinery needed for the radiography suite was listed. At first I could not imagine how the nascent company could possibly afford these very expensive items. Keith Chadwick recommended that expensive items of equipment, such as the operating table and X-ray machines, should be leased and not bought, so considerably reducing the capital we needed to raise to develop the hospital.

One of the medical committee members was Dr Anthony Kasassian, a consultant anaesthetist, who sent me lengthy notes on how to set up a hospital. This was most useful and included the following advice. "The first duty of the committee must be to vet the applications of those consultants who intend to take up shares and practise there (Euxton Hall Hospital). Doctors who want to buy shares as an investment but do not intend to admit patients should be excluded from the medical committee and only hold the same voting rights as ordinary shareholders."

A formal procedure to vet consultants applying to bring their private practice to Euxton Hall was immediately set up and controlled admission rights to Euxton Hall. "Kas," as Dr Kasassian called himself, also noted, "Consultants whose professional competence is suspect, and doctors who are known trouble-makers should be excluded from utilising Euxton Hall." More of this later; it was wise advice from a man who had studied his colleagues over many years.

The next task that fell to us was raising the funds. This was arguably the most difficult financial task the company was ever to face. Keith Chadwick had been busy, and the banks were willing to lend half the capital sum required, the other half being equity, with one proviso, those consultants who intended to admit patients to Euxton Hall should between them put up £60,000 in total from their own resources as proof of goodwill. Sixty thousand pounds seems a relatively small sum over thirty years later, but it was a significant amount of money in 1982. Raising this money would give comfort to the banks by indicating that potential users of the new hospital were willing to put their money where their mouths were. So if this money was not forthcoming, then the idea of a hospital could not be turned into reality. Plans were then made to approach and ask interested consultants to buy shares.

For the convenience of the prospective consultant users of Euxton Hall Hospital, a meeting was called for 28 September 1982 at 5.30 p.m. at the Bellingham Hotel. This hostelry was selected as it was conveniently situated opposite to the Royal Albert Edward Infirmary. The meeting was late starting but well attended. The small room rented for the occasion was crammed with people. Although inconceivable nowadays, the air was full of smoke from cigarettes and some cigars. Keith Chadwick introduced himself and informed those assembled about the plans for the new hospital, emphasising the excellent working environment planned. He then spoke about the necessary financial framework to develop the hospital. Potential users were then invited to buy shares. The meeting had gone well up to this point, but it now took a turn for the worse.

The first speaker from the audience stood up. It was Mr Donal Murphy, a consultant ENT surgeon, who announced that he had asked his solicitor to check with Companies House in London on the financial standing of Financial and Professional Services Ltd, which was Keith Chadwick's own company. The solicitor had reported that the annual statement of accounts for the previous year had not been lodged at Companies House. The meeting then went very quiet. Keith explained that Financial and Professional Services Ltd was a solid company, and the lack of recent accounts was merely an oversight. This did not prevent mutterings about "dodgy" businesses, and then someone mentioned the "Last Drop."

The name the Last Drop was repeated in several quarters, with further mutterings about losing all their money. The very name Last Drop had an unpromising ring to it. Those at the meeting who did not believe that the new hospital would ever be developed really got the bit between their teeth. They said that Euxton Hall was too far away from Wigan for their patients to travel there, and no direct bus route linked Wigan to Euxton. Mr John Stewart, a consultant surgeon, then said that the proposed hospital was too small to work and could not possibly survive, adding that he had a much better idea for a hospital. Further explanations by Keith Chadwick made some headway against this negative feeling, but the meeting finished with no apparent result.

Some consultants had real concerns and reasons for not putting their money at risk. The unpromising Last Drop was a village near Bolton where a few years before there had been plans to develop a private hospital. A number of consultants had parted with several thousand pounds, which they had lost, as the scheme became insolvent. While sympathising with their caution and desire not to throw good money after bad, it was pointed out that the Last Drop hospital scheme had been badly conceived. There was already an established and successful private hospital in Bolton itself, which would offer fierce competition to a newcomer. It had also been calculated that there was not the work for two private hospitals so close to each other. Last, the timing for building a hospital there in the late seventies was poor. It was an idea before its time. In comparison, the nearest competition to the proposed hospital at Euxton Hall was about twenty miles away and within the completely different catchment area of Preston.

Many consultants genuinely felt that their private patients would be unwilling to travel the seven miles from Wigan to Euxton for consultation or treatment, even though most people who were likely to use such a hospital would own a car. Mr Stewart's objection to the small size of the hospital was valid. Euxton Hall Independent Hospital as planned was to have only nineteen beds. This would make it the smallest private hospital in the country. With good management and busy consultant users, the directors were convinced it would succeed, but this was only a matter of judgement. We had taken a commercial view on its good prospects, and it was up to us to convince those who were sceptical that the project would be a success.

Keith Chadwick was not dismayed by these apparent difficulties, and to our delight several consultants did sign up and buy five thousand shares each over the next few months. The errant annual report for Professional and Financial Services Ltd was duly lodged at Companies House, confirming that that company was sound. More colleagues were persuaded individually over the next few weeks of the good prospects for a hospital in Euxton, with its wide catchment area and the potential to attract consultants not only from Wigan but also from Chorley and Preston.

Eventually twelve colleagues signed up and bought shares. The Conservative government of Mrs. Thatcher had arranged tax concessions to encouraging people to invest in new businesses. The banks were happy with the good faith shown by the consultants, so the necessary loans were forthcoming. Even the planning permission had been finally obtained. With these successes, the conversion of Euxton Hall into Euxton Hall Independent Hospital Ltd. was underway.

A bronze plaque was put up in the foyer of Euxton Hall Hospital, for all patients to see the names of those who had bought shares. There was a written disclaimer stating that each of these founding consultants, who were also shareholders, held no more than one percent of the equity. It was recognised by the consultants that patients had the right to this information. In all the years I worked at Euxton Hall, no one ever mentioned it, and being a shareholder never interfered in my professional relationship with any patient.

The names on the bronze plaque included Mr N. K. Maybury, Dr N. Naqvi, Dr C. M. Bate, Dr A. Kasassian, Dr I. W. Jones, Dr P. Reston, Mr M. Bell, Mr D. Murphy, Mr W. Balaero, and Dr D. Swinson.

The objection that patients would be unwilling to travel to the new hospital took some time to overcome. Taking a calculated risk of losing referrals, I moved my private practice, including consultations, to Euxton Hall Hospital on the day it opened and was pleased that my practice actually increased in size. I never advertised my services and left it to the assessment that general practitioners had of my work in treating their NHS patients.

I was the only consultant to see patients for consultation at the hospital during its first five years, but I was joined in time in the use of the hospital's single consulting room by Dr David Swinson, a consultant rheumatologist, who came on alternate Saturday mornings. After the early years, colleagues began to consult regularly, and by the midnineties four consulting rooms had been developed and were usually fully booked.

So the concern that patients would be unwilling to travel to Euxton Hall Hospital was unfounded. Over an eighteen-year period only one patient referred to me did not want to come into the hospital, asking me to operate nearer her home in Bolton. This I did not agree to do, explaining it was not satisfactory to have a single patient in a distant hospital, as I would not be able to see her daily and thus look after her postoperatively. Understanding my reasons, but anxious to be operated on nearer home, she went to seek a surgical opinion in Bolton.

Attention now concentrated on the conversion of the old hall into a hospital with all the associated building works. Another urgent task was the appointment of a matron. An advertisement was placed, and the six candidates who applied were shortlisted for interview. Mrs M. Williams was appointed. Mrs Williams was the second person to be appointed to the staff, the first being Mr Harry Barlow, the gardener. Harry had started working at Euxton Hall forty years before as an under-gardener and gave continuity with the past. I had been anxious that the gardens of the hall should not be neglected and allowed to deteriorate in the months before the hospital opened. Gardens that have run wild are difficult and expensive to restore. Harry not only maintained the gardens—the rhododendrons and azaleas were spectacular in the spring—but he was also a versatile and resourceful handyman and factotum, capable of carrying out multiple useful tasks. He had a good way with people. A few months later, Harry was to be found in the operating theatre as a porter, bringing patients to and from their rooms. What next? I thought and asked him jovially when he would start operating. Quick as a flash, he answered in his gruff voice, "They only have to show me once!"

Mrs Williams proved invaluable and worked diligently in preparing the new hospital for the admission of patients. This included the appointment of nursing and other staff. The board instructed that only a skeleton staff be appointed, with just enough nurses to run the hospital day and night when it first opened. At the same time a "bank" of nurses who were interested in part-time work was gradually built up. As the bed occupancy increased, nurses on the bank could be brought in as needed, and later, these nurses could be appointed to permanent posts. This worked well, and the turnover of staff was very low. This policy was adopted on my advice after learning from the experience of another hospital.

A large private hospital had opened a year or two before in Glasgow with enough staff to manage the hospital as though all the beds were occupied from the day it opened. When this hospital first opened, the bed occupancy was very low, which the directors had failed to anticipate. With the huge number of staff, including consultants, many of whom were on generous contracts, the financial burden was too great. This hospital in Glasgow went into liquidation due to staffing costs. We were determined to avoid this fate by implementing the policy outlined above. We were also fortunate in not having to employ consultants, as all our potential users were part-time consultants in the NHS and so self-employed. They would be operating at Euxton only on private patients referred by general practitioners to them personally.

On Tuesday, 19 July 1983, the first ten patients came to the hospital for consultations. It was the first time that patients had visited the hospital by coming to my first consulting session at Euxton Hall Hospital. All went well, and several patients were booked in for operations that August. Matron reported at a board meeting later that day that the bookings for inpatients for August would give bed occupancy of 15%.

These figures gave us all anxiety, even though it was known that the development of the hospital was under budget by £50,000. The hospital had cost £522,000 to bring it to readiness to admit patients, a quite remarkable achievement by Keith Chadwick and his team. Looking back over the years the amounts of money now seem small, but at that time it was a lot of money, and in spite of our optimism there was no guarantee of success.

In October, I reported to the medical committee that although the occupancy was disappointing, there had been the odd days when the occupancy had reached 85%. For a long time, I was in the habit of checking the occupancy figures every week. They always seemed low. However, the break-even figure for the hospital was just below 30% occupancy; steadily this figure was being achieved regularly and later surpassed with increasing frequency.

One of Dr Colin Bate's patients was the first to be admitted for any procedure, in this case an endoscopy. This was successful and gave all the staff confidence. The first admitted for an operation was one of my patients. The woman in question was of middle age and very jaundiced due to impacted stones in her common bile duct that were obstructing the flow of bile into the duodenum.

Elaborate preparations were made, including a trial run of the operation. This took place two days before her admission. The dress rehearsal covered all aspects of the operation, from sending the trolley to collect the patient from her room and bring her to the anaesthetic room. There, Dr Kasassian, my anaesthetist carried out a complete check of all the drugs that would be used on the day and included a dummy run on the anaesthetic machine, checking that everything worked and that everything that could possibly be used was available.

Then the trial moved from the anaesthetic room to the operating theatre. There instrument packs were opened and instruments handed out in the sequence that they would be used, thereby checking that nothing that might be needed was absent. After all the surgical instruments had been worked through, the radiographer brought the mobile X-ray machine, and we went through the process of taking operative X-rays without actually using films. The trial then moved to the recovery room and finally back to the "patient's" room, with a formal hand-over to the senior nurse. There were no hitches, and we were all confident that all would be well on the day.

When the great day arrived, the operation went according to plan, the gall-stones were removed from the common bile duct, and the X-rays taken to check that the bile duct was clear were of good quality. The patient returned safely to her room. She was discharged home ten days later with her jaundice fading and made an uneventful recovery.

Euxton Hall Independent Hospital was now truly open for work. Patients received the highest standard of care. It was always a pleasure to work there with cheerful and competent staff. The nurses tended to stay for years, giving great continuity of care. There is no better way to start a session than a cheerful greeting at reception. This applies even more to patients who can naturally be nervous. If their first contact in a hospital is pleasant, then they are much more likely to be put at ease. Euxton Hall Hospital was from the start a happy place to work.

It was during these early days after the opening of the hospital that it became apparent that there was a problem with the matron's management of the hospital. She had done invaluable work in getting the hospital ready to open. Unfortunately, she had great difficulty in managing bed occupancy. For example, if my colleague Mr Mervyn Bell had booked a patient to come into hospital on a Friday for an orthopaedic operation on the Saturday, Matron would not allow another patient to be booked into that same room earlier in the week, in case the earlier patient had not gone home. Great skill is needed in "bed juggling," and a clever ward sister can maintain high bed occupancy without having to cancel patients.

No amount of explaining, chatting, discussing, or remonstrating with Matron made any difference. Alas, this was a very important matter, for without someone with the requisite skill it was quite simply the case that the hospital could not succeed. Beds would be left empty when they should be in use, and the overall bed occupancy would never get much above the break-even level. Matron's dismissal was agreed by the board of directors as an unfortunate necessity at their next meeting. If the Matron had stayed in charge, there is no doubt in my mind that Euxton Hall Hospital would have gone bankrupt due to low bed occupancy, even when there were more patients who could be admitted. So with regret, she was dismissed.

The new nurse in charge was Sister Peck, an expert bed juggler. The occupancy soared, as she ably facilitated a steady increase in patient admissions. She remained in charge for some years, and when she retired she was replaced by Mrs. Bernie Dickenson, who had been senior sister for some years. Mrs. Dickenson was an excellent manager and liked to roll up her sleeves to be involved in nursing and teaching nursing, in which the hospital had begun to participate. She was one of the last of the nurse managers still capable of not only directing but also providing patient care personally, either in the NHS or private sector.

Within several months of opening, the hospital was admitting enough patients to break even and had become profitable within two years. As mentioned, I had been in the habit of looking in the admissions book every time I visited the hospital to see how many patients were admitted that day. I stopped that habit when it was no longer a hope but a reality that the hospital was running successfully, not just from a medical point of view but also financially. This was not only a great relief, but also a great pleasure to see. Board meetings, which had been ad hoc for the first eighteen months, settled into a two-monthly routine and still took place mainly in the evenings in my home in Standish. My wife provided supper for everybody and even sat in informally on some of the early meetings. Keith Chadwick ran the meetings very well, and they rarely lasted longer than an hour or two at the most, leaving plenty of time for general discussion. We had also gradually increased the number of new directors on the board.

The first addition to the original two directors was Mr John Lyons. Keith Chadwick and he had known each other for years. John was on the board of Keith's own company Financial and Professional Services Ltd. He was a chartered surveyor by profession and had excellent business acumen and a quite remarkable ability to find prime sites for development. Also Mr Charlie Brown, formerly chairman of a large building company in the North West who had backed the nascent company heavily with a purchase of 50,000 shares at the time when it was very difficult to find investors.

In 1984, as chairman of the board of directors, Mr Brown had declared that no dividend was payable that year and then privately bemoaned this lack of a dividend. I brightly said, "Charlie, you must take the long view," to which he replied in a quavering voice, "I've not got a long view." There was general laughter round the table. The following year the first dividend was paid, and Charlie was much happier. His knowledge of the complexity of the building trade was invaluable in advising the company how to produce an excellent hospital while keeping costs down. He was sadly right about not having a long view, as not long afterwards he died.

Further appointments to the board included Dr Nayyar Naqvi as the second medical member, an excellent colleague of mine also based at Wigan. He was a consultant cardiologist who built the cardiology services at the RAEI, developing a first class unit. Later, he was awarded a well-deserved OBE for services to cardiology.

Board meetings were always friendly. There was an air of excitement about them with so much going on. Nothing stopped the polite humour even in the most difficult of times. The board was ambitious that the hard-won expertise and knowledge gained by developing Euxton Hall Independent Hospital (EHIH) should only be a beginning of an expanding enterprise.

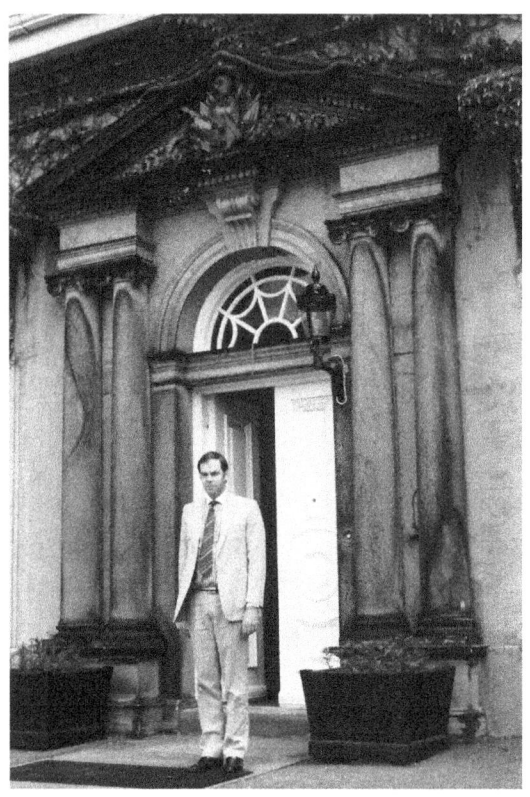

The author in front of the entrance to Euxton Hall Hospital in 1985.

Euxton Hall was bought with seven acres of land and had cost just under £200,000. The total cost, including the conversion of the hall into a hospital was only £522,000.00. This first of what eventually became Independent British Hospitals, opened on 26 July 1983, at an amazing price by any standards. The board took great pride that EHIH became, over the next few years the most profitable private hospital, for financial return on capital expended, in the country. No corners had been cut in developing this attractive building into an excellent hospital.

This paradox of high quality and low overall price was resolved by keeping all management fees within Keith Chadwick's own company. The hospitals were converted or built using the knowledge that Keith's firm had of developing hotels. Commercial suppliers were used for all fittings except the hospital beds, and this alone gave a great cost benefit. Another example was that all the kitchen fittings were bought "off the peg" from hotel suppliers at a fraction of the price that it would cost any NHS hospital. Amusingly enough, the first brochure produced for the hospital followed a hotel brochure format a little too closely by mentioning haute cuisine and fine wines!

Expensive medical equipment was either purchased second hand—mostly from bankrupt stock, but only the very best makes—or leased; for example the X-ray equipment, which was new. The operating theatre was bought as a module and then fitted neatly into the space in the operating theatre building complex that had been designed by my wife, Sara, and me! The non-executive directors received no pay or perks, although we did get to drink a glass or two of the "fine wine" at board meetings several years after the hospital opened—but not until it was a going concern!

A gap in the provision for private hospitals in towns across the country had been identified by the executive directors who had observed that the number of people medically insured had begun to grow rapidly in the early eighties.[1] The time was right and ripe for expansion. Now that Euxton Hall Independent Hospital Ltd (EHIH) had been successfully launched as a private hospital, it would be easier to approach banks, who would immediately take any proposal for new loans seriously; it would also be easier to find private backers.

Keith Chadwick and John Lyons formed a separate hospital services company in 1984, and in 1986 this new company became Independent British Hospitals Ltd (IBH) and was the management and development company for all our new hospitals. This company also held the management contract for Euxton Hall Independent Hospital from its opening. Then, to take advantage of cities and towns in Britain that we had identified as being under bedded for private healthcare, coupled with finding suitable sites in or near these locations, it was decided to develop four more hospitals immediately. These hospitals were to be situated in Preston, Southport, Carlisle, and Workington.

This new hospital group, North West Independent Hospitals plc, was separate from Euxton Hall Independent Hospital Ltd, of which I was a director. The expertise learned from the development of Euxton Hall was essential to these new hospitals, and they were brought into the fold a short time later.

Meanwhile the first development by IBH itself was a hospital at Stafford commissioned by Euxton Hall Hospital Ltd. Rowley Hall in Stafford had been a grand house, once owned by the Earls of Shrewsbury, but had fallen on hard times. It had been used as a school for a number of years. The cost of conversion to a hospital was contained within a budget of £1.7 million, and it opened on schedule for patients in September 1987. Thus Euxton Hall Hospital and Rowley Hall Hospital constituted another hospital group. It was very impressive that these hospitals had both been opened on time and within budget. The development of Euxton and Rowley Halls compares very favourably indeed to the inefficiencies and costs, and the time it takes for any build in the NHS at that time.

Late in 1987, IBH was involved in the formation of a third hospital group, called the Northern Independent Hospitals plc. Northern Independent Hospitals commissioned IBH to develop four hospitals. This history will get more complicated, and if the reader will bear with me there is a reason for including this information. If however exhausted by Euxton this and Northern that and IBH the other and how they all relate, you may prefer to skip the next few pages.

However, there may be a few whose interest is aroused by a history of the growth of a small corner of the health-care industry in the last twenty years of the twentieth century. This was still a time when the members of the medical profession were free to organise their own working lives. Private hospitals at that time recognised that consultant surgeons and physicians were their actual customers and so managed their business accordingly. After all, consultants could bring their patients to a particular hospital or not. It was the business of the hospital to provide the best possible working environment for the surgeons and physicians, and at the same time offer the safest possible environment and comfort for patients.

In 1986, IBH needed to raise £5.2 million under the Business Expansion Scheme[2] to fund the development for Northern Independent Hospitals. One evening, I joined a room full of people who had come to invest in the new company. By the time I arrived, several million shares had already been bought, and the atmosphere was electric as money poured in. I bought some shares myself. By the time I left for home, late that evening, most of the share issue had been sold. This was a stark contrast to the difficulty of raising the £60,000 from consultants needed to show the banks our serious intent and goodwill for the purchase of Euxton Hall and its conversion. All of these new groups of hospitals were developed by Keith Chadwick and his business partners, who were the executive directors of them all. IBH wasted no time in building the first hospital for Northern Hospitals Ltd at Washington in Tyne and Wear, which also happened to be the first built on a brown field site and the largest private hospital built in the North East. It was completed in under a year enabling the opening to take place on 23 May 1988.

The directors spent much time talking about the best way to raise capital for the further growth of the company. It was agreed that the various groups should, over time, be consolidated into a single company. This would make raising venture capital easier; a single company would hold all the existing hospitals and new developments. It then would also be large enough to consider an application to the London Stock Exchange for a listing.

Following this strategy, the first move was that in 1987 Euxton Hall Independent Hospital Ltd made a paper bid[3] for, and acquired IBH, which was Keith Chadwick's development and management company. Euxton Hall Independent Hospital Ltd immediately took IBH (Independent British Hospitals plc) as the company name for the merged business. So Euxton Hall Independent Hospital itself became a subsidiary of the new IBH. I had now become a director of IBH.

Within the space of five years, the company—having opened Euxton Hall Hospital in 1983 and Rowley Hall in Stafford in 1987— now also had the management business of the four hospitals it had built and continued to manage for North West Independent Hospitals plc, (Fulwood Hall at Preston, Renacres Hall in Southport, and small hospitals at Carlisle and Workington). In addition, the new IBH had a contract to build and develop three more hospitals for Northern Independent Hospitals.

After the development of Euxton Hall Independent Hospital, the raising of capital was never to be so difficult again. However, access to money is not the only problem that companies face. The executive directors, Keith Chadwick and John Lyons, were first class. Vince Sarsfield, who joined as the finance director, was from the same mould. As the business expanded, it became impossible for the initial directors to cope with the volume of work, and new appointments needed to be made. It became apparent that it would be difficult to find people of the right calibre, and two of these later appointees caused the company problems in different ways.

The first was a self-confident young man with excellent references. As he settled in it was apparent when talking to him that he was very busy. He seemed to be carrying a disproportionate burden for the company. He was well thought of in the early days. However, his expenses as presented to the board were excessive. This was most noticeable in the second and third years of his employ, when his expenses were huge. None of the other executive directors had claimed more than a tenth of his claims.

He had a penchant for fast cars and expensive meals, flying into Manchester Airport and hiring a Porsche to help him get about the North West in style. Samuel Pepys often used the phrase that somebody or something was "talked up." In his case, he talked himself up. Such people take care to make useful friends in high places. These friends give them full support, seemingly unable to recognise that they themselves are being used. While talking himself up to anyone who would listen, he was talking down his colleagues, especially his boss, in order to give the impression that he was carrying a disproportionate load and generally saving the company. The share options he had been given made his severance from the company a moderately expensive exercise.

The second was caused by a member of the administrative staff, who was appointed in the early nineties. I remember as yesterday his coming in late to a board meeting. When the agenda item labelled "operations" came up, he proudly announced that he had bought a private hospital in Manchester. My blood froze, and there was silence round the table. I had not heard that this purchase was even contemplated. If I had known I would have opposed the purchase because Manchester was oversupplied with private beds. Competition with established consultants in convenient facilities was inevitable, and so the hospital would be unlikely to generate the revenue expected.

It is interesting to trace the sequence of events that led to this state of affairs. When this hospital opened it was not used by many of the consultants who he had said would do so, resulting in fewer patients being admitted. Therefore the occupancy only reached the point of breaking even. This manager had spoken to all possible consultant users and thought that they said they would use the facilities, when they had only said they might.

Part of the art was to discover where consultants currently carried out their private practice and whether their existing arrangements were convenient geographically with good facilities and also for how long they had practised at that hospital. A well-established consultant who had been practising for years in a convenient hospital was very unlikely to move, whatever his protestations of interest. Such consultants should have been noted as unlikely users of the new hospital. It was necessary to attract new consultants or those who were inconvenienced for example, by only having access to an operating theatre at times that did not fit in with their other commitments.

These problems did not affect the company as a whole and Independent British Healthcare plc continued successfully, and was sold to Community Hospitals Group[4] in January 1998 with assets of £57 million, a turnover of over £37 million and a payroll of slightly less than nine hundred, of which more than half were nurses. The founding directors in particular took great pride that the company had come from nothing in 1982 to being the United Kingdom's fourth largest provider of private hospital health care as measured by the total number of beds. That we had provided direct employment for so many people also gave great satisfaction. As previously noted, the very first hospital, Euxton Hall Independent Hospital, was for many years the most profitable private hospital in the United Kingdom for capital expenditure. The policy of providing quality, both in buildings and medical equipment, was established and vindicated, with regular maintenance, renewal, and updating.

For fifteen years I was a director, first of Euxton Hall Independent Hospital plc, which eventually became Independent British Healthcare plc, and my close involvement in this exciting and rapidly expanding enterprise was not only interesting but also had other benefits. First, there was the sheer pleasure of working at Euxton Hall. I mentioned earlier that the first-draft plans of this hospital were produced within a week of my suggestion that Euxton Hall might be converted. This same pace was continued year after year with all the hospitals. I discovered that the power of a board of directors is immense. Once a course of action had been decided by the board, it was implemented without deviation or any change. Compare this with the NHS where it can take months for the simplest decision to be taken, and this decision can always be reversed by a higher committee, up to government level. In contrast, all IBH hospitals were built within contract for both time and cost. This was a magnificent achievement accomplished by the board of directors signing the developer's contract only when all specifications, detailed down to the last brick and bed-pan, had been negotiated by our quantity surveyor with the contractor. No aspect of the contract was then changed, and penalty clauses were included.

In contrast all contracts within the health service tend to wildly overrun—not least, in my view,—because people on each tier of the hierarchy think it is their job to be hypercritical of existing detailed plans. Therefore, they feel it necessary to make some change, often of a minor specification at a late date with ruinous consequences to cost and time. The proper role of these people is to oversee the contract and endorse it, only making changes if this has been improperly done.

The Public Finance Initiative for building NHS hospitals in the nineties was a prime example of these problems, in that not only did it cost a fortune, but the post-build service contract and interest were far too costly. This would never have been accepted if IBH was contracting the work. This contrast between IBH and the NHS in the modus operandi for commissioning and contracting building works was a great eye-opener, from which I learned a great deal. In addition, the directors of private developments have usually invested money in the enterprise and have an incentive to keep costs down.

I carefully managed the time consumed by being a director. One thing that I much appreciated about my co-directors was that they were willing to put in as many hours as I did. Eventually, by the nineties, the board meetings took place in different locations but usually at the accountant's offices in Preston in the afternoons. Since by this time board meetings were all scheduled at the beginning of the year I took a half-day holiday for each meeting, and by arrangement they hardly ever clashed with fixed NHS sessions, such as outpatient clinics or operating lists. If they did clash, I gave my apologies and was absent from the board meeting. In total in the average year I used about a week of my NHS holiday entitlement for my commitments as a director.

For eleven years (1982–1993) the non-executive directors were not remunerated for their input at board level. In 1994, the board decided that the chairman should receive £15,000 a year, and the other non-executive directors £10,000. So between 1994 and 1997, I received £10,000 per annum for being a director and in 1998 received £5,000 for loss of office when the company was sold. In retrospect, I know it was luck that the invitation was passed on to me to attend that cocktail party at Euxton Hall in early 1982, for which I thank my predecessor, Mr W. Weatherstone-Wilson (1915-2013). I am sure that if I had not attended, Independent British Healthcare PLC would have never have existed.

The role of a surgeon on the board, when that initial excitement of drawing architectural plans and playing a significant part in raising the magical seed money was achieved, was varied. It was essential to take an active part in the governance of the company, to give advice concerning medical matters. This included liaison when necessary with the local medical officer of health, who wanted to know exactly who would be allowed to admit patients and what the hospital would be doing. Licensing and inspection of private hospitals fell within the remit of the local health authorities in 1983.

Only consultants working for the NHS[5] were eligible to admit patients. There was no other career pathway in those days, and it almost always ensured a high standard of care was maintained. The local health authority came and inspected the hospital before opening and issued a licence for medicine and surgery to be practised there. Thereafter there were unannounced inspections on a weekday approximately every two years. These inspections were very strict. The health authority had the power to close the hospital. There were never any major problems, and minor ones were dealt with formally within six months to comply with instructions issued by the health authority. These were always reasonable, and the company always complied within the time scale laid down. In all, we had a very good relationship with the Chorley and the other Health Authorities. This initially entailed my attending a few meetings and writing letters, thereafter the matron of each hospital took on these duties.

Then there were discussions of all matters financial that all directors must take part in. These were very detailed, and I learned to read a spreadsheet. Beside this, there were important matters of policy pertaining to the relationship between a hospital and its clients. The hospital's clients were, as already noted, the consultants. It was the hospital's aim to provide consultants with the best possible working environment, with modern facilities and pleasant and comfortable surroundings for the patients. In this way everything was done to attract consultants to treat their patients in Independent British Healthcare Hospitals. The patients were referred by their GP to individual consultants by name.

However, from early in the eighties, a discussion was started by BUPA (British United Provident Association) with the management of all private hospitals to require that BUPA-insured patients be treated only at hospitals approved by BUPA. In itself, this did not appear unreasonable as all the IBH hospitals were recognised by BUPA. Later an idea was being pressed that GPs must refer their patients to an approved hospital, and in this case only a consultant who had been approved by BUPA would be entitled to see and treat those patients. Under this suggestion the patients would effectively become the hospital's patients, and the consultants would be invited by the hospital management to take on the care of individual patients. The result would be that both GPs and consultants lost their independence. This suggestion was an attempt to restrict the GPs' freedom to refer their patients to the consultant they thought would treat their patient best. I am pleased to say that while I was a director, the consultants and GPs remained independent, as I was able to keep these ideas and plans in check.

As soon as Euxton Hall Independent Hospital was opened, I left Fairfield Hospital, and from 19 July 1983 all my private practice (PP) was done at Euxton Hall Hospital. The practice grew, and by the end of 1985 approximately five hundred patients had been referred to me by their GPs in that year. Give or take a few tens of patients, this rate of referral remained constant for the next fifteen years. How this constancy in numbers continued was difficult to work out, as GPs left, retired, or died. In 2000, which was my last full year before retirement, the numbers declined slightly. I expected this trend of decline to continue due to the changing relationship between GPs and consultants.

The practice manager for PPs was my wife, Sara, who was extremely effective. We decided, when we arrived in Wigan, that if we were to run a successful practice we would abide by the three 'As' that I first learned about from Mr Brendan Devlin at St Thomas's in 1969 and noted in chapter two. Sara took all the telephone calls for referrals and made appointments for consultations. She also arranged, if requested by a GP as urgent, for me to carry out a domiciliary visit, even if late at night or at weekends. She could arrange these appointments or visits without needing to refer to me first. This worked well as the GP knew by the end of the telephone call what was arranged and could inform the patient or their family accordingly.

If patients tried to make referrals bypassing their GP, she politely directed them back to consult with their GP, and if the GP felt it was appropriate, to ask for a referral letter. One day I received a letter from the CEO of the Wigan and Leigh NHS Trust to let me know that a complaint had been lodged against me. The complainant had said that his time had been wasted by being made to consult his GP for a referral letter to me as a private patient. The CEO said he was letting me know as a courtesy, as my private practice[6] was nothing to do with him. My wife always explained to patients that seeing their GP first was in their best interests, because by consulting their GP, they would receive advice and know if the referral was appropriate. It was also of great importance that the GP knew what was happening. The complaint certainly raised a smile, as this was normal procedure.

References.

1. Between 1980 and 1990, the number of people insured with a private medical insurance company (PMI) increased from 3.6 to 6.6 million. There was little growth between 1990 and 1993, due to the recession, but by 1994, it was projected that over the next few years the number insured with a PMI would increase to nine million, representing 15% of the population. Quoted from "Admission to the Alternative Investment Market by Independent British Healthcare PLC 1995," registered number 2050024.
2. The Business Expansion Scheme was originally introduced in 1981 to give a tax incentive to those looking to invest in unquoted trading companies. It allowed capital losses to be offset against income tax and a reduced capital gains tax on capital gains. It was very successful in encouraging the building of new businesses.

3. In a paper bid, the shareholders of the company being taken over are given shares in the company taking them over, and no money changes hands.
4. Prospectus. Recommended offer by Granville and Co. on behalf of Community Hospitals Group PLC to acquire the share capital of Independent British Healthcare PLC. Shares must to be lodged with the registrars by 3.00 p.m. on the 6th January 1998.
5. Private practice as an NHS consultant was permitted by taking a part-time NHS contract, with reduction in salary, while maintaining continuity of care for NHS patients.

TABLE 11
The hospitals built/developed by Independent British Healthcare plc, from the opening of Euxton Hall Independent Hospital Ltd in 1983 to the sale of the company in 1998.

1982. Foundation of Euxton Hall Independent Hospital
Ltd (EHIH Ltd) with B.K. Chadwick
and N.K. Maybury as founding directors.
1983.Euxton Hall Independent Hospital opens.
1987. Rowley Hall Hospital, Stafford. Subsidiary to
EHIH Ltd.
1988. EHIH Ltd aquires IBH Ltd and takes the name
IBH Ltd. IBH Ltd had build/developed
and managed the following hospitals for North
West Independent Hospitals plc:-
1986. Fullwood Hall Hospital, Preston.
1986. Caldew Hospital, Carlisle.
1986. Renacres hall Hospital, Southport.
1986. Cumbrian Independent Hospital, Workington.
1989. IBH Ltd opened park Hill Hospital, Doncaster.
1992. North West Independent Hospitals plc aquired the
entire share capital of Independent British
Hospitals plc (formerly IBH Ltd). The board of
the new IBH plc becomes the board of directors
of North West Independent Hospitals plc.
N.K.Maybury is appointed to this new board.
1993. Northern Independent Hospitals plc aquires the
entire share capital of North West Independent

Hospitals plc. The board of directors of North West Hospitals plc becomes the new board of Northern Independent Hospitals plc. The Company now becomes Independent British Healthcare plc. &N.K.Maybury remains on the Board of Directors. The following hospitals had been built for Northern Independent Hospitals plc:-

1988. Washington Independent Hospital, Washington, Tyne and Wear.

1990. The Oaklands Hospital, Salford.

1990. Woodlands Hospital, Kettering.

1994. Northern Independent Hospitals becomes Independent British Healthcare plc.

1996. Independent British Healthcare plc is admitted to the Alternative Investment Market.

Additional hospitals built and managed:

1990. Kings Park Hospital, Stirling.

1991. The Tunbridge Wells Hospital, Tunbridge Wells.

1991. Abbey Park Hospital, Barrow.

1992. Carrick Glen Hospital, Ayr.

1993. Berkshire Independent Hospital, Reading.

1994. North Downs Hospital, Caterham.

1994. West Midlands Hospital, Halesowen.

1994. Victoria Park Hospital, Manchester.

1998. Community Hospital Group plc acquired the share capital of Independent British Healthcare plc.

Appendix

Case Histories

1. A family of multiple endocrine neoplasia (MEN I)
2. A case of infected aortic graft
3. A case of morbid obesity

1. A family with multiple endocrine neoplasia

The following case description illustrates decisions that needed to be made on clinical grounds alone. It also shows the range of surgery required.

In late 1980, a man of thirty, whom I shall call Mr Thomas, was admitted with dysphagia that had been increasingly troubling him for two weeks and had now resulted in a total inability to swallow—even water—during the previous twenty-four hours. Once rehydrated with intravenous fluids, he was submitted to a water-soluble barium swallow, which showed a complete obstruction at the lower end of his oesophagus. CXR showed no abnormality, and there were no other tests available that would be helpful diagnostically. It was not possible to see the cause of the obstruction with the rigid oesophagoscope, given the limited view obtained, nor was it possible to pass a narrow-bore tube through the obstruction, which was total. No other endoscope was available.

In keeping with current practice, an emergency exploratory diagnostic laparotomy was performed. A small hard stricture was found at the lower end of the oesophagus. Since cancer was the most likely diagnosis, and as the patient was unable to swallow, a lower oesophago-gastrectomy was carried out. The patient made a good recovery.

The histology of the resected portion of the oesophagus showed a benign ulcer surrounded with contracted and hard fibrous tissue. There was no evidence of cancer. In these circumstances, the most likely diagnosis was that the stricture was secondary to a gastrinoma, a rare tumour. The hormone gastrin normally stimulates acid secretion by the parietal cells in the stomach in response to a meal. A gastrinoma, however, produces gastrin in uncontrolled amounts, resulting in a vast outpouring of acid into the stomach, causing severe inflammation of the lining of the stomach and peptic ulceration. This is Zollinger-Ellison's syndrome[1] named after the two physicians who first described it. A blood sample from Mr Thomas was duly sent for serum gastrin assay. It was known that the assay result would not be ready for eight weeks, as this was the usual time it took to receive the results of hormone analysis in 1980.

Ten days after his operation, Mr Thomas started bleeding profusely from his stomach. The clinical diagnosis was that he must have developed a peptic ulcer in his duodenum or stomach. The bleeding was so profuse that he needed three units of blood to be rapidly transfused to restore his blood pressure. However, as the bleeding showed no signs of stopping, and since there were no investigations that might help accurately diagnose the site and the cause of his haemorrhage, the only course of action was to take Mr Thomas back to the operating theatre. When I opened his stomach, it was apparent that he had generalised and very severe gastritis and was bleeding profusely from the lining of his whole stomach.

These findings clinically confirmed that a gastrinoma must be the underlying cause. A detailed search did not reveal any obvious tumour in the stomach or pancreas. Since the stomach had been freed at the original operation, it was easy to resect the remaining portion of it.

The anaesthetist, Dr Wyn Jones, warned me that the patient was now in a very poor state and might not survive. However, the lower end of the oesophagus had to be attended to. It was not possible to bring a loop of small bowel halfway into the chest, so an oesophagus-to-small-bowel anastomosis was not possible, and in the patient's precarious state, a colonic interposition would have added to the patient's trauma. At this point, the sole objective of operating was to secure the survival of this young man.

Oversewing the lower end of the oesophagus alone would be certain to leak, however carefully it was done, because mucus and saliva would continue to be secreted and accumulate in it. Mr Thomas would certainly not survive any further complications. After careful consideration of the risks, I decided to continue operating and do the minimum to give Mr Thomas a chance of survival. This minimum was considerable, however. The operating started with closure of the duodenum and formation of a jejunal stoma for feeding purposes, as there would now be no continuity between his mouth and small bowel.

The abdominal wound was then closed. Mr Thomas was turned onto his side, and the chest incision from the original operation was reopened. Most of the remaining oesophagus was resected, leaving just enough of the upper oesophagus to bring it out as a stoma on his neck. To accomplish this manoeuvre the chest was closed, and a new incision was made on his neck. With careful dissection the oesophageal remnant was brought out as a stoma above his right clavicle. This operation, eight hours long, was a massive undertaking..

The good thing was that the bleeding from his stomach had been stopped within a few minutes of opening his abdomen by clamping the stomach preparatory to excising it, and there was minimal blood loss thereafter, allowing Dr Jones to stabilise him haemodynamically.

To my delight, Mr Thomas survived, and after a few days he was fed a liquidised diet by tube through his abdominal stoma. As he recovered, he started eating by mouth again, but of course any food immediately came out of the oesophageal stoma in his neck, which had a stoma bag placed over it to collect what had been eaten. As time went on, he ate what he liked, but he still needed to be fed a liquidised diet via the abdominal stoma as, of course, there was no connection between them.

Exactly eight weeks after sending the original sample of blood for serum gastrin analysis, the result arrived. It showed a sky-high serum gastrin, confirming the clinical diagnosis of gastrinoma and confirming that Mr Thomas did indeed have Zollinger-Ellison syndrome. The probably site of the tumour was the pancreas. The tumour is usually benign, and the only cells in the body influenced by gastrin are the acid-secreting parietal cells of the stomach. Since all these cells had all been removed by total excision of his stomach, no further search was made to locate a tumour or tumours.

A few months later when all had settled, I referred Mr Thomas to Mr John Bancowicz, consultant gastro-intestinal surgeon at Manchester Royal Infirmary, who very neatly interposed a part of Mr Thomas's colon between the oesophagus in the neck and his jejunum in the abdomen. This worked well, and gradually he was able to eat normally again. All these procedures proved to be the right course, as Mr Thomas was alive and well twenty years later.

The story did not end there, because in 1985 Mr Thomas's sister was referred to me by my colleague Mr Bill Richmond, our consultant urologist. She had been sent to him with kidney stones, which he had removed surgically, and she was found to have a raised serum calcium level secondary to hyperparathyroidism. I shall call this lady Mrs Almond and relate the continuing saga of this family.

On exploration of Mrs Almond's neck I found a single large parathyroid adenoma and excised it. Mrs Almond's circulating parathormone then returned to normal, as did her serum calcium. Most patients with this problem are cured and develop no further kidney stones. A rare complication of the overactive parathyroid is the development of a peptic ulcer, usually duodenal, which Mrs. Almond was known to have on admission with her other troubles.

The ulcer did not settle as expected, and as endoscopy was now routinely available, a gastroscopy was carried out, revealing nodules in the duodenum that were biopsied. These nodules proved to be part of an apudoma[2] a very rare tumour secreting a mixture of gastrin and glucagon. Since it was before the time of CT and MRI scanners, the only course was to proceed to a diagnostic laparotomy.

At operation, the pancreas was studded with discrete nodules from head to tail, many of these were over a centimetre in diameter. There was also no obvious evidence of pathology in the lining of the stomach itself, and so I immediately proceeded to carry out Whipple's operation, removing the whole of the pancreas with the duodenum. This was in January 1986, and Mrs Almond made an excellent recovery. She returned to work six months postoperatively. During her convalescence, she mastered her surgically precipitated type 1 diabetes.

All was well until 1988, when Mrs Almond again developed the symptoms of peptic ulcer in the stomach suggestive of Zollinger-Ellison's syndrome. By now a serum gastrin assay was back within ten days and showed a very high serum gastrin confirming a recurrance of Zollinger-Ellison's syndrome. Now, instead of immediately reaching for a scalpel, I approached the pharmaceutical giant Astra for assistance in acquiring their new drug Omeprazole, which acts directly on the acid secreting cells and inhibits the cellular proton pump to stop acid secretion. Omeprazole was then used on a trial basis only for treating patients with Zollinger-Ellison syndrome. The clinical trial had only just finished when I contacted them in early 1989, but Astra were very helpful, and Mrs Almond was duly started on 60 mg a day. The dose was rapidly escalated to 180 mg a day. At that dose the ulcer healed, and this was confirmed at endoscopy. She has continued to be controlled by Omeprazole since. It was now confirmed that Mrs Almond suffered from multiple endocrine neoplasia type I (MEN I).

This was still not the end of the story for Mrs Almond. She presented at a routine follow up in my clinic in 1993 complaining of severe headaches of several weeks' duration. Using an opthalmoscope, I found she had papilloedema in both eyes, indicating increased intracranial pressure. I rang our consultant neurologist, Dr Moore, who saw her later that same day and confirmed the finding of papilloedema and arranged an urgent CT scan that showed a brain tumour. A benign glioma was removed by the neurosurgeons shortly afterwards. She made an excellent recovery and was still alive and well when I retired in 2001.

Amongst Mr Thomas's and Mrs Almond's siblings, another brother had Zollinger-Ellison syndrome, and another sister had a parathyroid adenoma removed. They proved a most interesting family with MEN I. They were to be congratulated for their uniform good humour and fortitude shown over many years. I do not know the results of screening of the next generation of that family for this genetically inherited condition, but it was very important that this should be carried out. All the family were aware of the importance of screening, and before retiring I arranged appointments with a consultant endocrinologist for this to be done.

References

1. R. M. Zollinger and Ellison, E. H. "Primary Peptic Ulcerations of the Jejunum Associated with Islet Cell Tumours of the Pancreas." *Ann. Surg.* 142 (1955): 709–23; discussion, 724–8.

2. R. W. Spence and Burns-Cox, C. J. "ACTH-Secreting 'Apudoma' of Gall-Bladder." *Gut* 16 (1975): 473–6.

2. A case of aortic graft infection

In August 1994, a sixty-six-year-old man presented with a tender aortic aneurysm more than six centimetres in diameter, which I replaced with a synthetic graft. He made an uneventful recovery and was discharged ten days later.

One Thursday in October 1997, I was called as a matter of great urgency to the endoscopy room where Dr Colin Bate asked me to look down the endoscope he was holding to inspect the duodenum of a man admitted following a massive upper gastro-intestinal haemorrhage. When I looked down the eyepiece the duodenum was visible with a huge posterior ulcer with fresh blood around it. The main object that caught the eye was the edge of a Dacron graft in the base of the ulcer, which was violently pulsating, making the blood clot that was preventing further bleeding look decidedly fragile. The visible portion of Dacron had to be the upper edge of a tubular graft used to replace an aortic aneurysm. The patient's old notes had just been delivered to the endoscopy room, and I saw that the operation note was written by me, showing I had replaced his aneurysm three years before.

As it was a Thursday, my firm was on "take" for emergencies, and I had an all-day operating list that was proceeding at that very moment. I had left my registrar to finish the operation in progress, while I came to see what Dr Bate had found. Obviously this patient needed an immediate operation before a further bleed caused fatal exsanguination. Blood was already being cross-matched, and Dr Wyn Jones examined him and arranged his immediate transfer to the operating theatre. He was lifted on to the operating table without delay, the previous operation having just finished. The patient was anaesthetised, and in a long, difficult, and hazardous operation the old graft was replaced with a new one. The new graft was very close to the origin of the renal arteries, and it would not have been possible to carry out a different procedure—to close the aorta and ensure adequate blood flow to the renal arteries. The patient made a good recovery. Unfortunately the same patient was readmitted two months later having collapsed with a fall in his blood pressure. The signs on examination indicated an intra-abdominal bleed. At emergency operation, I found the bleeding was from the lower end of the graft where it was sutured to the right iliac artery. Due to the inflamed state of the iliac artery, it was closed after disconnecting the graft. Then to ensure blood flowed to the lower half of the body, a bifurcated graft was attached to the lower end of the aortic graft and anastomosed to the common femoral artery in each groin.

TABLE 12

ELECTIVE AORTIC ANEURYSM OPERATIONS
1991-1999

Number of operations	106	
Perioperative mortality	6	5.6%
Cause		
Cardiac arrest	2	
Generalised arterial thrombosis	1	
Haemorrhage	1	
Renal failure	1	
Septicaemia	1	
Non-perioperative mortality	2	
Cause		
Graft infection	2	
Time post operation	1	4 years
	1	5 years

Table 12. *This table shows the operative mortality in a series of elective abdominal aortic aneurysms replacements carried out by the author between 1991 and 1999. The patient discussed in this appendix*

was one of the two non-perioperative cases of mortality in this table. In both the cause of the complications leading to a fatal outcome was infection of the graft.

During the operation, alternative procedures were considered. One was to close the abdominal aorta below the renal arteries and then insert bilateral axillo-femoral bypass grafts to restore blood flow to the lower body. Again, because the renal arteries were at the very margin of the original anastomosis, I considered it unwise, especially taking the patient's critical condition into account.

Following this operation, the patient was very frail, treated in the intensive care unit and ventilated through a tracheostomy. Six days later a further exploratory laparotomy was needed to evacuate a large haematoma that had accumulated. The haematoma dealt with, inspection showed the new graft to be satisfactory. Gradual improvement followed, and several weeks later he was discharged and slowly regained his strength.

Two years later, in December of 1999, this unfortunate man died following a further catastrophic haemorrhage. He had been clinically well and living a normal life up to this final event. The underlying problem was a chronic infection of the graft. The difficulty of eradicating an infection in a graft is discussed in chapter 9.

In a huge US survey of 8185[1] operations on elective unruptured aneurysms, the mortality declined from 13.6% in 1980 to 5.6% in 1990. Mortality for ruptured aortic aneurysms was 49.8% with no improvement over the ten-year survey, and this is only the mortality of patients with ruptured aneurysms who reached hospital. To reduce mortality in the ruptured group, screening for abdominal aortic aneurysms[2] is now being rolled out throughout the United Kingdom and began in earnest in the first decade of this century. Those diagnosed with the condition are referred to specialist vascular units to monitor their aneurysm and if increasing in size to arrange for an operation as an elective proceedure with a low chance of mortality.

References

1. Katz, D. J., J. C. Stanley, and G. B. Zelenock. "Operative Mortality Rates for Intact and Ruptured Abdominal Aortic Aneurysms in Michigan: An Eleven-Year Statewide Experience," *J. Vasc. Surg.* 19 (May 1994): 804–815.
2. NHS Abdominal Aortic Aneurysm Screening Programme in men over 65. www.screening.nhs/aaa-england

3. A case of morbid obesity

In March 1986, a general practitioner asked me to see a morbidly obese patient who had suffered pulmonary emboli following a massive deep vein thrombosis and was now immobile. I did a domiciliary visit on this man, who was in his midthirties, to give my opinion on his suitability for a gastric bypass operation. The word bariatric was not in common use then.

My first experience of bariatric surgery was at the Middlesex Hospital, where the technique used was a small bowel bypass. The principle of this operation is to allow absorption of only a small proportion of the food eaten by morbidly obese patients, defined as being at least double their ideal weight. The operation defunctions 85–90% of the small bowel from absorbing nutrients. Technically it is not a difficult procedure. The upper jejunum is transected 20–25 cm below the duodeno-jejunal junction. Then the upper end of the divided jejunum below the duodenum is anastomosed to the terminal ileum a few centimetres above the ileo-caecal junction. The now-defunct end of the transacted jejunum, 20–25 cm below the duodenum, is closed. This enables the natural small-bowel secretions to flow down the bypassed jejunum to enter the caecum. All anastomoses were hand-stitched.

At Leicester in 1997, a different operation was being used. The "stapled banded gastroplasty" was technically possible only because of the advances and reliability of stapling devices. Here the principle is to make a very small pouch out of the upper portion of the stomach where it joins the oesophagus, so separating it from the main body of the stomach. This was accomplished by using two stapling devices and a silastic ring round the opening of the false pouch into the remainder (greater portion) of the stomach. On eating the pouch distends, stimulating the vagus nerve to transmit a message of fullness to the brain, which in turn inhibits the sensation of hunger. Unlike the small-bowel bypass, which is fool-proof, the banded gastroplasty can be cheated. One patient cheated by heating chocolate until very soft and then swallowing it. In this state it will slip easily through the new upper gastric pouch. Before being offered surgery patients had to attempt to lose weight by other means, such as eating less, having the jaws wired to prevent eating of solids, and last, by consulting a psychiatrist.

I met Mr Hindley at his home. I noticed that he was sitting on an armchair that he totally overlapped and hid from view. He was surrounded by a ring of toffee papers, and the box from which they came was empty. He was a likeable man, easy to talk to. He informed me that as a young man, at his peak, he had weighed eighteen stone (114.3 kg). He took a sedentary job, which by chance was close to a chip shop, of whose products he freely availed himself. He told me he weighed 46 stone (292.1 kg), which was later confirmed in the hospital. A few years before, a "health-food" firm had offered him £10,000 to lose ten stone (63.5 kg). Unfortunately, his determination evaporated after losing nine and a half stone. He then returned to eating seriously and rapidly regained all the weight he had lost. He had also had his jaws wired together several years ago, which had not stopped him taking a high-calorie liquid diet through a straw. In addition a psychiatrist had been unable to help. After careful evaluation, I offered him surgery.

The technical problems that had to be overcome before operating were considerable. A standard operating table was too narrow for such an enormous man, who would literally overhang both sides of the operating table and pose a real risk of rolling off. Postoperatively he was so heavy that only a team of people would be able to move him. In discussion with Dr Wyn Jones, the patient's consultant anaesthetist, it was decided that Mr Hindley must get onto the operating table by himself before his anaesthetic to avoid his needing a lift. While he was asleep under the anaesthetic the operating table must be safe and antistatic so diathermy could be used. Once the operation was over, his operating table must also double as his bed, where his postoperative nursing would take place. Until Mr Hindley had fully recovered from his anaesthetic he would need his position to be changed every two hours to prevent pressure sores from developing. Last, he must be able to get himself off the bed into a chair within twenty-four hours of the operation.

The solution was to make alterations to a King's Fund bed, which was strong and three feet wide (91.5cm). It could be pumped up and down, and its width ensured that there was no risk of the patient rolling off. Boards were placed under the mattress to prevent sagging. The mattress was itself sewn into an antistatic rubberised cover, and on top of that went a fireman's blanket, used to catch people jumping off buildings, which had strong handles at short intervals all round its circumference. Then an under-blanket was placed on the fire blanket with a sheet on top. The hospital works department made a strong metal bar that was securely fitted to the frame of the bed above his head. This was high enough, when covered by sterile drapes while operating, to enable Dr Jones and his assistant to have access to Mr Hindley's head and thus his airway. This bar was also strong enough and high enough to have chains connected to two retractors fixed to it. These retractors placed in the abdominal incision lifted the weight of the abdominal wall with its thirty-centimetre-deep layer of fat, so making access to the abdominal cavity possible, enabling the surgeon to work on the abdominal organs. In average-size patients, these retractors are held by assistants but this was impossible in a case such as this due to the sheer weight of his abdominal wall. I had a long discussion with the patient and emphasised how he must help us, especially by getting out of bed on the first postoperative day, to which he readily agreed.

On the appointed day in 1986, Mr Hindley climbed onto the bed-cum-operating table and was wheeled down to the operating theatre. Dr Jones was preparing to administer the anaesthetic when two senior hospital managers entered the surgeon's room saying that they needed to talk to me urgently. They said that the operation must be cancelled, as it wasn't safe to operate. I asked them why they had come to this conclusion, and they said they thought that the hospital would not be covered legally if anything untoward should happen. They thought the size of the patient and the makeshift operating table were the main points. Certainly Mr Hindley was the largest patient I had operated on, and I believe he was at that time the heaviest patient ever operated on in the United Kingdom.

I told the managers that a great deal of thought, care, and work had gone into the preparation for this operation. I had taken the decision to operate with a fully informed and consenting patient. He understood the balance of risks with the possibility of immediate problems during the operation and postoperatively. These hazards were to be weighed against the probability of an early death due his obesity and recurrent deep vein thrombosis if he did not have the operation. As a surgeon, I was used to balancing risks. I told them that there was no such thing as an operation without risk. However, doing nothing would carry a greater risk for Mr Hindley, and as with all my patients, I would take full responsibility. I informed the managers that the operation was going ahead. With that they left, and I heard no more about it.

A few minutes later the operation started. After the skin incision the deep fat layer could be split by traction on either side of the incision. This reduces bleeding but also displays the rather beautiful lobulation of the deep layer of fat that is clearly seen in these cases. The liver was large, turgid, and not malleable due to fatty infiltration. In addition the gall-bladder was chronically inflamed and full of stones. In spite of good retraction, the volume of fat in the abdominal cavity, coupled with the weight of the abdominal wall bearing down, meant it was impossible to manoeuvre the stapling instruments that are integral to the upper banded gastroplasty operation. Under these circumstances, for the patient's safety it was apparent that the only feasible operation was a small-bowel bypass. Before starting that, a cholecystectomy and appendicectomy were performed. The rationale for this was that in the morbidly obese it is notoriously difficult to make a diagnosis in the event of the patient developing peritonitis, or even recognising peritonitis, as examining the abdomen yields no useful signs due to the thick fatty mask covering it. The small-bowel bypass and other procedures were uneventful.

When Mr Hindley was awake, he was taken to the intensive care unit. Postoperative care was discussed with the sister in charge of the ITU and the nurse delegated to look after him. The nurse was about eight stone in weight, so I left written instructions that in the unlikely event of Mr Hindley rolling off the bed, she was not to try to prevent it, on the principle that an eight-stone person would be injured or worse while trying to prevent such an event happening to a fortysix-stone person! After seeing Mr Hindley settled in the ITU, I returned every two hours after mustering a gang of any ten willing persons to be found nearby—doctors, porters, and a few nurses—to man the fireman's blanket, so the patient could be safely turned and attention paid to potential pressure areas to avoid bedsores. This was done through the night, and by the next morning he had already started to drink fluids. We had previously discussed his convalescence. A very large armchair was placed beside the bed, and with only guidance, he slowly sat up and got off the bed and into the chair and later rose to walk a few steps. His postoperative recovery was uneventful, and he was discharged home a few days later. He was a very good patient.

Mr Hindley was monitored in outpatients and his weight loss was impressive while he continued with a good diet. Between June 1986 and December 1988 the weight loss was 18 stone (114.3 kg). In the first nine months of this period 15 stones (95.2 kg) were lost, and in the next nine months he lost a further three stones (19.0 kg). He was then lost to follow-up until six years later, when he appeared in A&E with an unrelated condition. The young doctor who saw him weighed him to find he was 25 stone (158.8 kg). The doctor suggested that he should consider losing some weight (not knowing his previous history) and was amazed to be told he had had a small-bowel bypass operation and had already lost 21 stone (133.3 kg). I last had news of Mr Hindley in December 2008 when Mrs Alison MacDonnell, the secretary to the anaesthetic department at Wigan, sent me paper cuttings showing that my former patient was well and slimmer than ever, weighing in at 17 stone (107.9 kg).

Table 13
Weight Change post small bypass operation

		Stone	Kilograms
12/06/1986	Date of operation.	46	292.1
08/10/1986	Weight at follow up.	37.3	236.9
05/11/1986		36.6	232.4
06/03/1987		31	196.9
09/09/1987		29	184.1
15/12/1998		28	177.8
06/12/2008		17	107.9
	Total weight loss to 2008		**184.2**

Epilogue

As a new consultant general surgeon at the Royal Albert Edward Infirmary in Wigan in 1980, my remit covered the whole gastro-intestinal tract, some aspects of thoracic surgery, biliary, pancreatic, paediatric, breast, endocrine, trauma, vascular, and acute abdominal surgery. In addition, I offered a special interest in gastro-intestinal and vascular surgery. I was sorry that the opportunity to carry out emergency neurosurgery, in which I had taken an active part both at Warwick Hospital and the Leicester Royal Infirmary, ceased. Urology, which I had learned under John Marsh at Warwick Hospital, was removed from the ambit of general surgery while I was working at the Middlesex Hospital and while I was at Leicester Royal Infirmary (1977–1980), the first consultant urologist was appointed there.

This broad canvas of work I much enjoyed (ch10/table 10). The first change was in the middle of the eighties, when a new colleague, Mr Richard Harland, was appointed as a consultant general surgeon with a special interest in breast surgery. At that time women with breast conditions were encouraged by the media to seek the advice of a specialist. This stimulated GPs to send most of their patients with these problems to Richard. He was an excellent general surgeon who found that the range of his general work was significantly curtailed by the sheer volume of referrals of patients with breast disease. The reduction in referrals to my firm of women with breast conditions did not reduce my overall workload, as there was no shortage of other patients to be seen, but by 1984–1985, the number of mastectomies my firm were carrying out noticeably decreased. Then in the midnineties another consultant breast surgeon was appointed and it was then that breast surgery virtually disappeared from my repertoire (table 10). The new appointee was the first surgeon who did not participate in the general surgery emergency rota, not having had a general surgical training. Now, super-specialisation was beginning to have an impact.

Next to super-specialise in the early nineties was paediatric surgery. For over ten years, I and my registrars had operated on babies with pyloric stenosis. Every few weeks, a baby with this condition was admitted and usually operated on in the evening as an emergency, being anaesthetised by one of the three consultant anaesthetists who had the expertise to manage these babies. Over these years the operative success rate was 100%. I then noticed that our consultant paediatricians were now referring all these babies to Pendlebury Children's Hospital in Manchester as a matter of policy. It was salutary to observe how rapidly the surgical—and especially the anaesthetic—expertise to look after these babies was lost at the RAEI.

In 1999 by agreement with colleagues, I stopped receiving new vascular surgery referrals from GPs in order to make room for a new consultant surgeon dedicated to vascular surgery to be appointed. The resultant fall-off in vascular surgery can be seen in chapter 10/table 10. On my retirement in 2001, I was replaced by two more surgeons, an upper gastro-intestinal surgeon and a colorectal surgeon, and the thyroid work was taken over by the ENT surgeons.

The reasons for other radical changes in the training and practice of surgery were driven by the advance of technology and the counterintuitive desire to replace the apprenticeship with more modern teaching methods.

My memoir attests to the great satisfaction achieved from the old ways of practice. There was the pleasure of operating over a very broad range of competence, together with the clinical freedom to control all aspects of professional life, knowing that the role of management was to provide the best facilities for good practice. However, there was no doubt that the apprenticeship training could be haphazard and sometimes unsatisfactory for some trainees. Moreover, while it was possible until 1999 to be working to a high standard across a very broad field, this was becoming more difficult with advances in knowledge and treatment. The rapid evolution of medicine was driven especially by the revolutions in electronics and innovation in instrumentation. Thus the practice of surgery was changed from an art and science, to the application of science and technology to surgery.

So the old ways could not last, but some of the consequences of the changes have been seriously detrimental. Management have unbalanced the practice of surgery by directing it, instead of providing the best environment for patients and for surgeons to practise, leading to dissatisfaction amongst many surgeons and patients. Targets set by governments can result in perverse priorities and can lead to inevitable game playing by management. For example, corridors with patients lying on trolleys have been designated as wards to fulfil the targets of reducing the time patients have to wait before being admitted. Clinical priority for operations has been overridden by management to keep within waiting-time targets. This means that patient's whose ailments are not favoured by being within a target, but have a serious condition, have their treatment delayed so targets can be fulfilled. In this way surgeons have lost the freedom they had over their professional lives and concern for their patients tends to be overridden.

The passing of the days when an individual patient was known to the firm throughout their stay in hospital is serious. It is compounded by the EU Time Directive, with its forty-eight-hour week, resulting in the necessity for surgeons to work in shifts to give twenty four hour cover. This results in the loss of the continuity of care which used to be given by firms, including consultants, working nights and weekends. These changes have resulted, on some occasions, in poor cover by senior doctors at night and a reported increased mortality among patients at weekends. It has also created difficulties for our future generations of surgeons to gain adequate experience.

There is also another matter which must be mentioned, which is the burden of medical litigation. This has now grown year by year to reach huge proportions in both volume and cost. This latter has reached several billions of pounds a year to the NHS. Even though the profession has resisted, it has led to defensive medical practice on many occasions and is a grave psychological burden to individual practioners when sued vexaciously. The downside is that investigations are sometimes no longer carried out solely on the principle of only being ordered if the result may change the treatment for a patient; to also being ordered to protect against litigation. All this is at significant cost to the service.

The direct control of budgets by doctors ceased as long ago as 1974. There had been little discussion in public, but with the shortened training, I believe that the profession will probably have to arrange itself as is done in some countries on the continent. That is to appoint, in each hospital, a senior practising surgeon to be the chief of staff, with all other surgeons, de facto, subordinate to him or her and to be directed and supervised in their work. This person must remain a clinician and not a manager. This would create a surgical chain of command giving the new chief of staff equality with senior management. It would, unfortunately, finally recognise that the days of all consultants having the satisfaction of reaching the top of their professional tree with freedom of practice may be over.

I am confident that the new generation of surgeons will continue to advance the science of surgery and fully accept and welcome the huge advances in the treament of diseases, as well as the necessity for change as inevitable.

I was lucky to have had the pleasure and privilege to be a general surgeon at the end of the twentieth century, before the golden age of the general surgeon finally ended.

Index

Abbreviations

Anaesthetist	anaes
Anatomist	anat
Cardiologist/Cardiac	card
Chief Executive Officer	CEO
Company Director	Dir
Consultant	con
Doctor of medicine	DM or MD
Euxton Hall Independent Hospital	EHIH
Fellow of the Royal College of Anaesthetists	FRCA
Fellow of the Royal College of Surgeons	FRCS
Fellow of the Royal Society	FRS
Fellow of the Zoological Society of London	FZS
Gynecologist	gyne
Haematologist	haem
Independent British Healthcare plc	IBH
Leicester Royal Infirmary	LRI
Middlesex Hospital, London	MH
National Health Service	NHS
Orthopaedic surgeon	orth
Past President RCS	PPRCS

Birmingham Accident Hosp, 36

Black, John. PPRCS con surg. 24, 129-130

Black, Sir James (1924-2010). FRS Nobel Laureate, 69

Blower, Anthony. MD FRCS con surg. RAEI, 121, 122

Board of directors EHIH, power of, 142, 160-161

Boughdady, I. FRCS surg reg. RAEI, 125

Brown, Charles. Chairman EHIH, 153

Burge test, 61-65

Business Expansion Scheme 1981, 157

Camel, injury by, 98-99

Cannabis, 21-22

Cardiac tamponade, 80-81

Carter, J F Bolton. FRCS con surg. LRI, 81, 112

Casualty Officer, StTs'sH, 20-24

Chadwick, Keith. CEO IBH, 142, 143, 144, 148, 152, 155, 157, 158

Chloroform, x

Cholecystectomy, 109, 110, 150

Christopher Home, Wigan, 138

Chui, Paul. FRCS reg. RAEI, 90, 123, 140

Cimetidine, 69

Cogwheel, RAEI, 93

Colonic cancer, screening, 114-120

Colo-rectal surgery, 10, 17, 28, 30, 38, 49-50, 114-120

Consultant, contract, xi

Consultant, status and responsibilities, xii, 93, 157, 163, 188

Continuity of care, 11, 20, 23, 24, 27, 45, 123, 129-130, 151, 187-188

Cowan, Dr Maxwell (1931-2002). PhD Fellow of Pembroke College, Oxford anat. 1

Crick, Dr Francis (1916-2004). OM FRS Nobel Laureate, 6

Cyriax, Dr James (1904-1985). MD con physical med. StTs'sH, 23

Davies, Prof D V. (1911-1969). FRCS FZS Prof anat. StTs'sH 24-25

De Bakey, Dr M E. (1908-2008). American surg. 31

Pavlov, Ivan Petrovitch (1849-
1936). Physiologist, 55
Pay, 16
Peck, Mrs. SRN Sister-in-
Charge EHIH, 152
Pembroke College, Oxford,
1-6
Pepys, Samuel (1633-1703).
Diarist, ix, 159
Perutz, Prof. M. (1914-2002).
Nobel Laureate, 3
Pneumothorax, tension, 35, 39
Poole, Dr. con path. 3
Prakash, Dr reg. WPH, 17
Private practise, 138-166
Professional status of sur-
geons, xii, 188
Prosector of Anatomy, 24-25
Prostatectomy, Millin's, 29
Psychiatric hospital, 38-39
Pyloric stenosis, surgery, 186

Reed, Dr Peter. FRCP con phy.
WPH, 18
Registrar's training, 122-127,
128-129
Reston, Dr P. con radiologist
EHIH, 147
Richmond, W. FRCS con urol.
RAEI, 172
Road traffic accidents,
32-37,104-105

Royal Albert Edward
Infirmary, Wigan (RAEI), 87-
133, 138
Rugby league, 99-100

St Thomas's Hospital, London
(STs'sH), 7-19
Sarsfield, V. Dir IBH, 158
Savage, C R. (1915-2004).
FRCS con surg. WH, 26, 31
Screening for colonic can-
cer, see colonic cancer
screening
Seat belts, 27, 34
Shafy, T. FRCS surg reg. RAEI,
123
Shouldice, Dr Edward.
Canadian surg. 82
Siney, Barbara. SRN ward sis-
ter RAEI, 88
Slack, Sir William W. FRCS
con
surg. MH, 44, 47-49, 51
Smoking, 144
Smyth, V. FRCS surg reg.
RAEI, 126
Spina-bifida surgery, 30-31
Spleen, operations, 28, 34,
102-104
Specialisation in surgery, 83,
96, 105, 136, 185-186

www.ingramcontent.com/pod-product-compliance
Lightning Source LLC
Chambersburg PA
CBHW051644170526
45167CB00001B/323